The SHORT Road to Health

7 Easy Lessons for a Longer and Healthier Life

Table of Contents

The Story

Introduction

Thank You

John Donne once said, "No man is an island." No truer words were ever spoken, and that is why I would like to thank some key individuals who helped make this book possible.

I would like to first thank my mother and grandparents. When I was a young kid growing up in a small fishing village in eastern Canada, I was acutely aware that we did not have the finer things in life. However, those humble beginnings and down-to-earth cooking allowed me to become the man I am today. I personally believe that the foods we eat at a younger age, when our genetics are still developing, are the most crucial in our lives. I grew up on turnip greens, wild berries, and seafood. Foods that were cooked by my loving mother, as opposed to prepackaged by large agribusinesses. As you will read in this book: *Nutrition is the key to health.* My early memories were gloriously nutritious. Not only did we eat healthy, but we would also run, play, hike in the clean air and swim in clean cold waters. Life in eastern Canada fills my mind with pleasant memories of simpler times, which were a great foundation for growth into adulthood.

I would like to thank my wife and children. I am a highly driven person and, to external people, I can often seem frazzled or excessively busy. I never personally feel the stress of this busy life, but how others see me may differ from my personal evaluation. It takes a special family to endure ambitious personalities. *I* have been blessed to have such a family, thank you so much. I love you all.

It has been said that we walk on the backs of Geniuses. I did not discover the research that is discussed in this book. Others, more intelligent than I, have dedicated their lives to uncovering the truth about the human experience. All I have done is connect the dots and observe trends with my patients. Without the work of these people, my work could not be possible and for that I am forever grateful.

I would like to make a special thanks to my editor, Kassie Reep. My English grammar has always been terrible, which is a deficit that I have always been somewhat ashamed of and have covered up by stating that I am a "man concerned with content." I love to teach and see the moment when a student grasps the content. This flash of light has been a big part of my life and what keeps me enthusiastic about teaching. Nevertheless, my grammar continues to "suck," and my content could not be understood without the diligent, skillful mind of Kassie. Thank you so much.

Lastly, I would like to thank Bob Stovall for taking on the graphic art of the cover, book formatting, and liaison to the publishing company. I am extremely busy, and without your help, this book would have taken me five years to get printed. Thank you.

Dedication

I dedicate this book to all of my family, friends, and patients who have left the living before their time. I pray that you are in a happier place and that your souls are free to fly. You will be forever missed.

About Dr. Dennis Short

Dennis was born in a small, quaint fishing town in Newfoundland, Canada. Due to the death of his father at a young age, his family was forced to live very cheaply. When a family has little money, they learn to survive on what is available. If a lower-income family lives in the southern Unites States, they might eat grits and alligator. Living in Atlantic Canada, Dennis's family lived close to the land; eating cabbage, turnip, carrots, wild berries, moose, and ample amounts of seafood. Junk food and highly processed foods were a rarely enjoyed luxury.

Hard work and the fresh Northern climate allowed Dennis to grow into a healthy and strong individual. Once in college, he struggled with finding the proper career direction that suited his personality and skill set until he discovered chiropractic. The philosophy of chiropractic states that the body has an innate ability to heal itself. It was this truth, along with his personal belief in wholesome food that allowed Dennis to become a successful chiropractor. He has continued his studies on the art of living well by not only studying research, but also observing thousands of patients in his chiropractic practice: "Too often people rely on what research tells them to do without observing how things really happen in the real world." Dennis personally believes that the art of being healthy and living a long life exist where science and practicality meet.

After treating thousands of patients from diverse, socioeconomic backgrounds, Dennis is acutely aware of the trials that some individuals endure, and for that reason, he is very pragmatic about the struggles patients have on the path to getting well. He asserts: "It can be difficult to turn your life around and get healthy, but people can do anything they put their minds to. If you want it badly enough, anything can be accomplished with the correct attitude and information." Dennis is committed to people and to their quest to discovering health. This book is a shining example of that commitment.

You don't have to feel tired, grumpy, unhappy, and sick. There are things you can do to change your life for the better. Start today, and discover the healthy, vibrant person that resides inside of you. It is there, all you have to do is use the information in this book to bring out the healthy you.

"Each year most people feel worse than they did the last. If you change your life, you can be one of the few who will be better next year. It is not about how fast you reach your goals, it is about being on the right track."

Dr. Dennis Short D.C.

The SHORT Road to Health

7 Easy Lessons for a Longer and Healthier Life

She tipped her head towards my shoulder, not fully placing her weight on my body as if she was not sure she could fully trust my sincerity. I felt her tears trickle from her cheek onto my shirt while her hair tickled my cheek. The tickle almost made me sneeze, but with every inch of my willpower, I fought the urge. Her mascara-stained tears ensured that my white shirt would never come clean, but I dared not say a word.

I could feel the heaving of her body as she sobbed uncontrollably against my chest with shallow, rapid breaths. I tried to imagine the thoughts that must be racing through her mind. I'm sure it was impossible for her to have any coherent thought pattern. How could anyone think straight under such pressure? Her emotional outburst was laden with an impossible mix of confusion concerning her loss and overwhelmed frustration with regards to her future. What would be her financial limitations? How would she deal with the trials of raising children by herself?

All of her questions came tumbling out with spit and tears in one broken, stuttering utterance, "Why did this have to happen?"

I wasn't sure if she wanted an answer or if the question was even directed towards me. Perhaps it was rhetorical or maybe it was directed towards God.

We had been friends for many years, and even though I felt extremely comfortable around her, no amount of friendship could prepare someone for her situation. Normally a fix-it-myself type of person, I felt increasingly uncomfortable. Even still, I reminded myself that this situation was not about me. But how does one console a thirty-two-year-old widow?

My friend, her husband, had just passed away from cancer. It started as a skin lesion that spread to his nervous system, eventually killing him. The whole town was in shock. He had served as a pillar of our community, everyone had loved him. In fact, a person couldn't help but love him. He recognized the good in everyone and always pointed to the silver lining in every dark cloud. The world would definitely be a little darker in his absence.

Looking back down at his grief-stricken wife, I debated what to say. I did not want to sound patronizing, especially since I could not possibly understand what she was going through. Nor did I want to belittle her struggle by pretending I had some great revelation for her. Feeling like my hands were tied, I finally conceded to offering her the line of support everyone seems to default to when trying to comfort the inconsolable.

"I don't know what to say. I can't make any sense of it all and I don't want to upset you by trying. I know you must have a million things running through your mind. I do want you to know that I'll be there for you, to listen and help you in anyway possible."

I tried to voice my generic response with as much tenderness and compassion as I could muster, but the truth was that these words were odd for me. I am very opinionated and at that time, I had a very blunt opinion in regards to why her husband had died. When a thirty-five-year-old man dies of cancer... there has to be something wrong. God did not screw up that much. But I couldn't say that to my friend's bereaved wife. Besides, what would it accomplish at this point? If I had owned a time machine to go back a decade or two, perhaps I could have made a difference. Voicing my opinion now would just piss her off. No one likes to be kicked when they are down and I was not about to be the one doing the kicking.

Instead, I just sat there with her head on my shoulder, her tears continuing to soak into my already damp shirt. We stayed there for over an hour until her tears just couldn't flow anymore. The salt had stained her light skin and created a red irritation under her eyes. A person can only cry so much before their body will shut down the production of tears. This of course, did not mean that my friend's sorrow had abated. It just meant that once her body had recuperated, she invariably would start crying again.

"Is there anything you would like to talk about?" I asked with some apprehension. Though I doubted she had gained any clarity over the past hour; I wanted to understand what was going on inside her mind, hoping against hope that I might be able to help.

I have been a fixer all of my life. If someone is hurting, confused or needs help, I have always been the one to call. Some people have told me that my fixing tendency is a common trait that can be a great detriment to the male population. There are times when some people just want to vent without asking for help. But this concept is hard for me to understand. I had been sitting with my friend not fixing anything for over an hour and I could feel my natural instincts rapidly swooping in. I wanted to know more.

"He was my soul mate," she proclaimed. At first I thought she was about to start crying again, but her tear ducts just couldn't handle the strain. I knew then... regardless of how capable I might have been to fix the various facets of her struggle, our conversation was bound only to wandering in grief-confused circles. Only time would eventually sever the rope that had her brain knotted to her lost, devastated heart.

Sadly, situations like these are becoming more and more common. I am not naïve to the facts of life. I am acutely aware that all living things must die, but in this day and age, it seems as though people are dying younger.

I believe, and the American Medical Association would agree with me, that 85% of all human illnesses are preventable. The other 15% of illnesses can be contributed to genetic deficits and accidents. Our lifestyle choices of excess stress, bad diets, dehydration, and lack of exercise are killing us. I have no idea if my departed friend would still be with us if he had maintained a healthier lifestyle, but I can say that if he had made better choices, he would have had an 85% better chance of preventing his cancer.

With that in mind, I have decided to write this book with the hope that some people would obtain a clearer picture of health. Health is not a difficult concept, but scientists and the general population act as though it is getting more and more elusive. This book will give you some easy, cost-effective methods to preventing disease, increasing the quality of your life, and possibly preventing an early death.

To accomplish this goal, it will not be necessary for you to cut out all of your favorite foods or to exercise for five hours a week. In fact, not only is it not necessary, such habits can be very destructive to your health.

The material in this book is derived from reading hundreds of articles and books on health, as well as treating and closely observing thousands of healthy and unhealthy patients. Because of the knowledge my education and chiropractic practice have afforded me, I consider it my responsibility to share this information with the world to help prevent 85% of American diseases—as well as to potentially help you not die young.

"The future depends on what you do today."

Mahatma Gandhi

Introduction

Even though I am only forty years old, I already have had two friends my age and younger die. Both of these individuals had cancer that they fought and tried to manage, but ultimately they died. They were cut down in their prime, both happy, vibrant people who not only added value to my life, but also to everyone with whom they came into contact.

Since I have been in private practice, I have had many patients even younger than myself die from a variety of conditions ranging from obesity, diabetes, strokes, heart disease, and cancer. Again, I am well aware that death is a part of our human experience, but why so young? When I was a young adult, my generation seemed to think that death was only something that old people had to deal with. Now, all age groups are developing deadly conditions and having to worry about life after death.

My friends that have passed away left behind a spouse, children and loved ones all wondering how this could possibly happen to them. While life is funny sometimes, it is certainly not a joke. Although the average life expectancy is increasing in the Westernized world, our younger populations are being afflicted with more and more chronic diseases. Some sources even say that the life-expectancy age is dropping for the next generations. In my career, I have treated twelve-year-old kids who are already morbidly obese and suffering the early stages of diabetes. They are cutting their lives short but remain too young to fully realize the repercussions of their actions.

We are constantly bombarded with television and internet advertisements promoting new diets and weight loss programs, yet we continue to be historically fatter and sicker than any of the generations before us. Our culture admonishes us to run longer and harder to stay healthy. Physical trainers order us to exercise so much that we feel like we will pass out. Yet despite these new lifestyles, our generation is not living healthier or longer. What is the answer? How did we get here? And how will we get back to our natural state of health?

I personally believe that we are fatter and sicker than ever, because we have stopped thinking. We would rather have a scientist tell us what is okay to eat than to use our own minds. Ironically, scientists are more confused than ever, in regards to nutrition, but refuse to admit their ignorance. If they admitted their ignorance, the American populace would loose confidence in their abilities, consequently stripping them of their ability to manipulate the food industry and earn the food corporations billions of dollars.

Case in point, many scientists believe that we don't live on whole food as much as we live on the nutrients within our food. They believe that it is not the food itself that adds value to our existence, but rather the nutrients and vitamins composing the food. Although this method of reductionism seems logical at first glance, it assumes that we don't need to eat whole foods to obtain the raw nutrients residing within our food. Hence, though we have heard our grandparents chide, "Eat your carrots because they are good for your eyes," we are now instructed: "Take your vitamins that contain vitamin A because vitamin A is good for your eyes." Is this true, or is there something bigger in carrots that make them good for eyesight? Something more than just vitamin A?

The food industries that make pizza pockets and instant meals may have added vitamins and minerals to them, but does that make them healthier than steak or squash? Surprisingly, whenever I ask a patient, which is healthier—pizza pockets or butternut squash—they always get the answer right. Butternut squash. Whenever I ask a pregnant mother, which is better for her baby—formula or mother's milk—she always answers correctly. Mother's milk. If we are so smart on an individual basis, why do we as a general population make such poor food decisions?

The exercise dilemma is equally confusing. Recently I was in an airport and noticed a group of women who were each wearing gold medallions around their necks. So I had to ask them, "What do the medallions represent?"

With obvious pride, one of them explained that each of them had earned a medallion for finishing a half marathon. For you readers who don't know anything about running, that means that each woman ran a total of thirteen miles. Knowing this fact, I decided to look around at as many of these ladies as I could to attempt to profile them and their various body styles. From my observation, the ages of the women appeared to range from twenty-five to fifty with various heights and races. But regardless of the wide range in ages, heights, and races, each woman had one thing in common with the next: excessive abdominal fat. Every single woman was bulging at the belly—in spite of their deceivingly thin legs and arms! Many call this body shape a muffin top.

My point is that we have all been told that running is great for us and that if you want to lose weight, it is one of the best ways to do so. But my eyes don't lie. These women were not thin; nor were they the poster representation of a healthy, long-distance runner. At some point, we have to open our eyes and realize the truth: Excessive cardiovascular exercise does not work for weight management. This is not to say that running is not good for your heart and lung health. It is to some degree. But overall, long-distance running can have some detrimental effects and is not a good weight management tactic.

Staying healthy is not difficult, but we do need to start thinking and stop listening to others. Diet soda will not help you lose weight. If it did, diet-soda drinkers would be thin. Are they? That has not been my observation. Low-fat food is not healthier than regular food. If it were, people eating a low-fat diet would be thinner and healthier. Are they? I've not made that correlation. Obviously, cutting calories is not a way to lose weight and keep it off.

Let me explain it this way. The heaviest patient I have treated in my practice weighed about 450 pounds. She tells me that she has tried everything to lose weight but has found nothing that works. In my opinion, she obviously has not tried everything. If she had, she would be thin. Nevertheless, when I questioned her eating habits, I noticed that she eats far less calories per day than I do. At first thought, most people would blame her obesity on her genes, assuming that she simply is genetically predisposed to that condition. But as I dug deeper into the details of her lifestyle, I discovered her problem. She does not eat many calories, but when she does eat them, she consumes them all at one time in the course of one meal. Care to guess which meal that is? If you guessed the last meal of the day, you would be correct. As a society, we have gotten used to our evening meal being our largest meal of the day. From your body's perspective, it is the worst time of day for you to consume the majority of your calories.

Knowing this, I had talked to her until I was blue in the face about how she needs to eat more calories more often throughout the day, but it was too late. She had been brainwashed to the point of no return when it comes to thinking that if she eats less calories, she will lose weight—never mind the fact that she is now heavier than she ever had been in her life since she decided to stop eating three meals a day. Why is it that she can't see her problem? Because she has been told a lie for so long that she now believes it.

When your body is starving for nutrients and calories, your metabolism will decrease, and you will store most of your calories as fat. The key to effective weight loss is to keep your metabolism high throughout each day, allowing it to consume your calories rather than store them. But we will talk further about this topic in the upcoming lessons on food and exercise. This is just a taste of what is to come.

For now, I contest that getting healthy and staying healthy is not as difficult as many people would make it seem. With few exceptions, being healthy is our natural, God-given state. We only lose our health and vitality when we make poor decisions that ultimately deviate us into the realm of disease.

As I stated earlier, the AMA contends that 85% of all diseases are preventable, and this book was created to assist you in that prevention. Of course, not all diseases are preventable. No doctor would be silly enough to claim that he or she had the cure for all human ailments. There will always be a person who follows a healthy lifestyle yet still gets ill and dies at a young age. Equally, there will always be those people who do everything wrong but live to be old. These exceptions defy logic, but exceptions are also a fact of life. We cannot plan for abnormalities; we can only deal with averages.

Bearing that in mind, I have had many patients whom I have convinced to quit smoking, abusing alcohol, or lose weight in an effort to alleviate some of their symptoms and assist them in experiencing better health. This book will not deal with those particular physical problems or addictions. No intelligent person thinks that smoking or drinking excessively is beneficial to his or her health. I do not need to insult your intelligence by writing a book about the importance of smoking cessation. There is no way that you can be healthy if you smoke a pack of cigarettes a day, just like you cannot walk in perfect health if you are 100 pounds overweight. Having one or two cigars a year will not shorten your life neither will being 10 pounds overweight kill you prematurely. Let's use some common sense here. Enjoy the pleasures of life, but don't shorten your life by enjoying them daily.

Moreover, as a chiropractor, it would give me no greater pleasure than to tell you that the key to your personal health lies within receiving chiropractic manipulations. But that would be a lie, and I will not tell a lie. It is true that your brain and nerves control all of the activities necessary for your body to function healthily. It is also true that interference with this functioning can be detrimental. Still yet, even though spinal-joint manipulation has been proven to remove neurological interference at the spinal level and ultimately allow for better communication between your brain and body, it is not the most important factor in being healthy.

This book was created to highlight the most critical factors affecting human health by listing those factors in order of importance from greatest to least. Surely improving any category of wellness will help you feel better and possibly prolong your life. Realize that true health is only actualized by improving all of the categories listed in this book. I have tried to write with plain, easy-to-understand English. Doctors are notorious for speaking with complex terms that only confuse patients. Hence, I have designed this book to be a very easy-read and it is kept short on purpose. I see no need to complicate the topic of health anymore than necessary. Health is not elusive; it is our natural state of being. It is not difficult to stay healthy, so let's not complicate it.

"You don't have to cook fancy or complicated masterpieces – just good food from fresh ingredients."

Julia Child

Lesson 1

Is My Food Keeping Me Alive or Killing Me?

In the past, food looked like food. An apple appeared to be an apple; strawberries, potatoes, and meat looked and tasted exactly how you would expect them to. But today, food comes in cans, microwaveable dishes and easy-to-prepare containers that only require adding water or popping in the microwave. That is, of course, if you decide to dine at home at all. The ingredients of these convenience meals bear little resemblance to actual whole food of days gone by. Most of the time, we have no idea what is in our food, and until recently, we haven't bothered to ask.

Now, as increasing numbers of the population have gotten sick, the wiser consumers among us have started to question the integrity of our food, asking questions like the following: Do we need to have hydrogenated fats in our foods? Do our bodies actually require all of the preservatives and dyes placed in our food to survive or to properly digest food?

More and more, healthcare professionals are realizing that these extra ingredients added to our food could be one of the major causes of sicknesses and potentially even premature deaths. If this really is the case, which I believe it is, then the food you eat is probably the most important factor to living with health. As the old adage goes, you are most definitely what you eat. Here's an example.

Not too long ago, I was at a restaurant and I picked up a packet of honey with the intention of making my dry chicken more palatable. Before I opened the packet, however, I got the urge to read the label on the back. To my surprise, the sticky liquid inside was not really honey at all. Instead, the list of ingredients revealed that the substance inside actually consisted of high fructose corn sugar and preservatives. Only 7% of the substance was actual honey! This is ridiculous when one considers that real honey is one of those wonder foods composed of all natural sugars that rarely spoil. Why, in the name of God, would anyone try to recreate honey from non-honey sources with the intention of trying to get it to taste like honey? The whole concept seems flawed and grossly unhealthy.

The above honey example is just the tip of the iceberg. I have seen blueberry muffins without blueberries and strawberry yogurt that contains no strawberries. Most of the time you are not eating what you think you are eating. So I have to ask: Are we better off today with all of these processed foods? I think not.

We have entered a time when we cannot trust the front label on anything. After all, the front label on my "honey" package said that there was really honey inside. Thus, if you want to start living healthily, you must learn to be a label-reader—and I don't mean the front label. I mean the back label.

When I read the back label on a certain package of food, I am less concerned with the percentages of fat, carbohydrates and protein as I am with the list of ingredients. Legally, ingredients have to be listed based on the percentage of their total contents. If high fructose corn syrup is the largest constituent in a certain product, then it has to be listed first, the second largest ingredient listed next, and so on.

The World Cancer Fund states that women have a much higher risk of getting cancer when they eat processed foods. To prevent diseases and to live longer, the key is to eat items with very few ingredients and only items whose ingredients you are familiar with and know. You may have no idea that propylene glycol (which is in many salad dressings and other processed foods, is really the scientific name for anti-freeze. In order to eat healthily, you don't have to. You just need to use your common sense. If you don't know what propylene glycol is, simply refuse to buy or eat products that list it as an ingredient. Point blank, if it is not food, you shouldn't be consuming it. It is not necessary for you to know what red dye number 4 is or why silicon dioxide is found in your popcorn seasoning. Rather, just be smart and stay away from unknown ingredients.

I am often asked about the benefits and risks of sugar substitutes. In my mind, they are all evil. Tricking your body into thinking there is sugar in your food when there actually is not can prove to be a dangerous activity. When your taste buds tell the brain there is sugar on the way, your body prepares for the carbohydrate onslaught by manufacturing and secreting insulin. However, because there is no sugar present in sugar substitutes to actually deliver the carbohydrates, dangerously low blood sugar can result—not to mention a heightened appetite, which is counterintuitive to why you were consuming those sugar substitutes in the first place. Interestingly enough, the low blood sugar that sugar substitutes can create in your body is similar to the high and low blood sugar swings experienced by diabetic patients, whose results can be even more severe.

Moreover, there are many adverse side effects attributed to using sugar substitutes. These can include the following: headaches, irritability, fibromyalgia, neurological problems, digestion, and immune system dysfunction. Now obviously, not everyone will get these symptoms, but even still, I personally don't think tricking the body into tasting a laboratory-derived sugar is a smart idea in the long run. There are many dangers with consuming sugar products and far more with consuming sugar substitutions. My recommendation to you is to not consume any sugar products, but if you have to choose among them, I would encourage you to take the calories from honey. I will explain to you why.

Most sugars are made from fructose and glucose. Between the two, fructose is more destructive. Table sugar (sucrose) is 50% glucose and 50% fructose. In contrast, high fructose corn syrup is 55% fructose and 45% glucose. If you would like to have a slightly better alternative than table sugar, try using honey. Although the concentrations of fructose and glucose in honey may vary depending on the different flowers from which the bees got the honey, on average it consists of 52% glucose and 48% fructose. This is not a significant improvement, but it is better—especially when you consider that honey also possesses other added benefits in its ingredients, such as vitamins, minerals and some antioxidants, with the darker honeys ranking higher. Added sugar products are not necessarily good for you, but at least honey is a better choice.

Let me break it down even further. When you eat sugar (a blend of fructose and glucose), the glucose is metabolized and absorbed into all of your body's cells, but the fructose goes straight to the liver. Once within the liver, the fructose is converted into triglycerides, which can cause fat deposition and, ultimately, fatty liver disease. Of course, this process is made even worse when food companies change a food product's main ingredient from sugar to high fructose corn syrup. Even though high fructose corn syrup only has slightly more fructose than regular white table sugar, you can't afford to have that excess since the fructose will be converted into triglycerides.

In short, the more chemical additives, dyes, and garbage that exist in our foods, the more our liver and kidneys need to eliminate these foreign molecules, placing a large strain on these organs. Excessive strain can cause organ failure or a toxic buildup of these chemicals, causing your system to clog and mess up your metabolism. If this happens, it is likely that you will become unable to effectively process fats, which could ultimately lead to obesity and heart disease.

Likewise, while low-fat, pre-made meals that you simply pop into the microwave might be convenient, they are loaded with chemicals. Perhaps you initially thought you were doing something healthy because the meal claimed to be low-fat, but the truth is that high-fat foods are not the culprits that are killing us. Rather, it is the refined sugars and preservatives that are making us fat and causing us to die.

To combat this attack on my health, I make a point to eat whole ingredients. When I buy bananas, I know that the only ingredient present in that food product is banana, just like I know that squash is made of squash and chicken consists of chicken. When you cook with these whole ingredients, you don't have to be as concerned with whether or not you are eating garbage.

That is not to deny the fact that many items in the produce section have been sprayed with large doses of pesticides and many meat items contain steroids and antibiotics. Surely these preservatives and additives can be a big concern, but I have less anxiety about this problem than I do with eating fast food or instant foods from your grocery store. Why? Because you can minimize these problem ingredients by washing your fruits and vegetables well before you eat them. Moreover, you can buy organic produce and steroid-free meats. Personally, I choose to buy all of my meats from local farmers and have them butchered locally. That way, I know that my meats are steroid and antibiotic free.

I also grow 90% of the vegetables that my family consumes in my own garden, thus ensuring the least amount of pesticides. That being said, I am aware that not everyone is capable of living my lifestyle, but the honest truth is that you don't need to in order to be healthy. Instead, just make an attempt to buy local vegetables from farmers' markets and steroid-free meats whenever possible.

Switching gears a little bit, you might have noticed that wrapped within this first lesson of eating real, whole foods is the aspect of cooking. The practice of cooking is becoming more and more foreign to modern, better-off civilizations that are concerned with convenience. Instead, children have grown accustomed to eating takeout pizza, Chinese food or processed canned ravioli. Many have lost the joy of cooking and see it as an unnecessary task. To counteract this destructive paradigm shift, please re-learn how to cook. Make it a family affair and get the kids involved. Teaching kids at a young age the importance of cooking will prevent them from falling into the average rut of eating junk food and getting sick. The health of our children is one of my biggest concerns because I see so many sick and obese children in my office. Children are easily programmed and if you teach them to cook at a young age, they will think it is normal. However, if you never cook and teach them to eat fast food each day, they will think that is normal. Old habits are hard to break; the best way to break a bad habit is to never start it. Let's take a greater responsibility for our kids' health and by doing so, make our country healthier. I see no better place to start than with our children.

Please understand me. I am not naive to the busyness of the average, American life. Moms and dads run from work to soccer practice and piano lessons. They believe that they are lucky to eat at all, let alone cook a meal for their families. But some simple planning and setting of priorities can easily cure this problem. Indeed, rather than worrying about your children growing up more cultured, encourage them to grow up healthy by allowing them only one extra-curricular activity after school with the condition that it does not interfere with dinnertime. For if you are doing so much that you can't eat healthy, you have your priorities a little mixed up and need to re-evaluate what you are spending your time doing...especially since you now know that today's children are dying younger.

A way that I have learned to save time when it comes to cooking is by utilizing my weekends for preparing large amounts of food so that I can save it for meals during the rest of the week. For instance, on the weekends I might freeze chili, soup, and lasagna so it can be simply heated later. Doing this has allowed my son and I to cook together on Saturdays or Sundays and has simultaneously given us great father-son time. He is learning his importance to me and also the value of eating well. When he gets older, I am positive that he will look back on these special times together with fond memories.

Your Unique Dietary Needs

A few years ago, Dr. Peter J. D'Adamo wrote a book entitled *Eat Right 4 Your Type: The Individualized Diet Solution to Staying Healthy, Living Longer & Achieving Your Ideal Weight.* The premise of the book suggests that people's blood types predispose them for specific diets that are optimal for their health and weight. When it was released, I was happy to see this type of book become popular because, for the first time within diet and weight-loss literature, authors and readers began to recognize the fact that not all people can eat the same type of food and be healthy. We are obviously not all the same, so why did we assume for years that we could all eat the same things and live healthy lives? There is a large genetic variation in the human species, and to believe that what is healthy for one person is also healthy for the next is ludicrous.

At the same time, I also believe that Dr. D'Adamo's book over-simplifies individuals' diet possibilities. We each possess millions of unique genes and for that reason; I believe that millions of different healthy and unhealthy diets could exist. The key to optimal health is *to* identify the diet that complements all of the subtle, unique intricacies of your own genetic make-up. Albeit, the process of discovering the perfect diet for you might be difficult, I believe that the rewards far outweigh the work in the end. Let me explain why.

Your genetic code is unique to you. No one on Earth ever has been or ever will be like you. You are one of a kind. Some of your genes produce the enzymes that *assist* you in properly digesting your food. Because of your genetic originality, these enzymes (in addition to your stomach acid) may be unique to you. Amazingly enough, your gastric juices are more unique to you than your fingerprints. They are a unique combination of stomach acid and gastric enzymes. Even if you and I had similar enzymes in our gastric juices, the concentration of our specific enzymes would likely varry, thus adding to our individual uniqueness. For this reason, I believe that you should have a specific diet that caters to your specific genes, gastric enzymes, and digestion capacity. Surely you are starting to see why there really is no one diet that "fits all."

For example, if you consume milk containing lactose without concurrently possessing the gene that codes for the enzyme lactase, you will not be able to fully digest the milk or any of its by-products. Instead, your body will react against the undigested lactose by creating inflammation within your gastrointestinal tract.

This process of reactionary inflammation has been understood for many years with regards to milk and a few other food products. This is the case for a lot of other foods. For indeed, any and all foods work the same. If you don't have the appropriate enzyme to degrade a certain type of food, it will cause inflammatory gut disease. However, inflammation in your gastrointestinal tract will not stay just there. The gastrointestinal tract has miles of blood vessels that will carry the inflammation throughout your body, causing inflammatory problems in many other tissues. It could trigger the inflammatory cascade into your arteries, resulting in excessive blood cholesterol and arthrosclerosis. Or it might spread to your joints and afflict you with inflammatory arthritis. Researchers and authors of *The Great Cholesterol Myth* assert that: "Acute inflammation hurts, but chronic inflammation kills." They go on to report that chronic inflammation can cause conditions such as Alzheimer's disease, obesity, arthritis, diabetes, neurodegenerative disease, heart disease, respiratory disease, liver or kidney failure and even cancer. The possibilities for disease due to food intolerance are endless. The key to preventing these diseases is not the proper use of drugs, but rather the prevention of chronic inflammation.

Some people have attempted to prevent diet-related inflammation by attempting to lower their cholesterol. However, the authors of *The Great Cholesterol Myth* tell us based on their research that such efforts are not the appropriate way to decrease inflammation in the body. According to them, inflammation can be likened to a fire in the body and cholesterol to the body's firefighters. Clearly, in their estimation, cholesterol is not to blame for people's inflammation-related conditions. Rather, they are proposing that when you attempt to decrease inflammation in your body by lowering your cholesterol levels, you simply are keeping the fire of inflammation burning. Such habits are what cause degenerative diseases, especially heart disease, and that is why I think this chapter is the most important lesson in this book if you really want to prevent disease and not die young.

That being said, the discovery of which foods are good for you and which ones are detrimental can be like searching for *a* needle in a haystack. It may take years for you to discover your true genetic identity, but I believe it is a must if you wish to live a long and healthy life.

The Elimination Diet

Let's get right to it and look at the best way to discover your perfect, genetic diet. We will use the process of elimination, a procedure that I have all of my clients perform in my weight-loss program. I will teach you the same process I teach them.

Before you start eliminating foods, you need to establish a baseline that consists of your weight and biographical dimensions for future comparison. For the weight portion of your baseline, just weigh yourself and record your weight.

To attain your biographical dimensions, use a tape measure to measure around your neck, biceps, chest, belly, hips, thighs, and calves, being sure to measure each leg and each arm, not just one of them. Afterwards, add up all of the measurements. Their sum equals the biographical dimensions part of your baseline.

Now you can begin the elimination process. Start by eliminating all dairy, wheat, eggs, corn, and soy products from your diet for one month. This means that for one month, you may eat any fruits, nuts, meats or vegetables that you want, with the exception of corn or soy products.

When that one month is up...weigh and measure yourself again. Compare the data you retrieve with your original baseline. If there is a difference between the two sets of data, it is very likely that you have discovered some of your individual food sensitivities. Amazingly enough, during this process when you remove a food product that you are sensitive to or cannot fully digest, you may loose 20 pounds and ten inches.

But the process of elimination cannot end with comparing measurements. Regardless of variance in measurements or weight, you need to continue to test for food sensitivities to dairy, wheat, eggs, soy and corn products by slowly adding them back into your diet. For instance, you can add dairy back in by drinking a glass of milk or eating some ice cream. If you actually do have sensitivity to dairy, you probably will get quite sick with possible bloating, gas, or diarrhea. Conversely, if you do not experience any adverse symptoms or gain back any inches in your measurements, you will know that you have no sensitivity to dairy and can eat dairy products for the rest of your life without wondering whether or not it is causing inflammation and slowly killing you. After 3 days start adding back in the next food item until you have discovered all of your food intolerances.

In addition, please note that you may experience symptoms denoting food sensitivity that are not physical. For example, you might experience mood swings, anger, depression or trouble concentrating. Oddly enough, the most common symptom that my patients have described to me is the feeling that their skin is "too tight" or "crawly." These symptoms are equally as important as the others and should be considered when attempting to narrow down your specific food sensitivities.

Again, only when you re-enter a food category back into your diet and experience no symptoms will you know that your body is capable of properly digesting that food product without causing any inflammation. The most common foods people generally experience sensitivities to include the following: dairy products, wheat and its various forms, eggs, soy and corn products. Nevertheless, in the process of trying to find your unique gene diet, you should not overlook any food in the process, and here's why....

I have a friend who is sensitive to garlic, while I myself have intolerance for cucumbers. Surely cucumbers are healthy for most people, but to my surprise, not for me. When I eat them, I start to feel bloated and struggle with excess gas production. Both symptoms serve as signs to me that I cannot digest cucumbers properly. If I insisted on eating them, despite these warning symptoms, I would create within myself a chronic inflammatory gut problem, which in turn could invoke a plethora of different diseases. So, keep eliminating different foods, and continue to pay close attention to how their re-admittance back into your diet is making you feel.

At this point in this lesson, it would be wise to warn you that when you first do an elimination diet, you likely will think that you are starving. In fact, you may consume 3,000 calories of fruits, nuts, meats and vegetables in a day yet still feel hungry. You need to know when this happens that you are not calorie-deprived, nor are you starving. What you are experiencing is a withdrawal process that is occurring because your brain is used to getting simple carbohydrates on a regular basis. Hence, feel free to eat as much as you like as long as you stay within the bounds of your elimination diet. You can rest assured that these cravings will pass in four to five days.

This is also a great point in the lesson to warn you that many of the foods that commonly cause inflammation in people lurk in hidden places. For instance, dairy can be found in many different places. It can be found in bread, cereals, potato chips, sauces, and flavorings. Often, it will have different names in these products like milk solids, milk powder, butter, buttermilk, cream, lactose, whey, and casein. All of these ingredients are either milk or derived from milk and have to be completely eliminated while undergoing the elimination diet. You need to be diligent about this elimination process. Many people try to cheat the process by contesting, "I don't have very much." To that I respond, "If you had an allergy to bee stings, how many bee stings would be okay?" The answer is obvious. None!

Therefore, in order to really succeed at the elimination diet, you must get use to reading labels to check for places where eliminated foods might be hiding. Corn can be found in the form of high fructose corn syrup or cornstarch, while wheat might be concealed under the disguise of names like wheat flour, bleached flour, enriched flour, durum wheat, semolina flour, or gluten. To help you avoid these disguised foods, I have compiled a list of food products in **Appendix C** that you should avoid during your elimination diet.

I will tell you firsthand that an elimination diet is not easy and that if you do not do it correctly, you will be wasting your time and making your life difficult for no reason. However, if you choose to do the elimination process correctly, you will attain the keys to a proper diet for you, which will make you feel better than you have felt in years.

Just recently I had a participant in one of my weight-loss classes experience great success with the elimination diet. When she started my weight-loss program, Julie was sixty-five years old and had suffered many sicknesses all of her life. She was overweight by about 60 pounds and had come to me in desperation because she had tried numerous diets to lose the excess weight without any of the diets proving successful. Discouraged, she admitted to me that even if she had lost some weight with the diets she had tried, she quickly gained her weight back once the diet was over. She was hoping that my program would be different and that I would be able to help her. So like always, I decided that she should discover and deal with her food intolerances first by way of the elimination diet. After only two weeks, she had lost 11 pounds just by eliminating dairy. When we tried to introduce it back into her diet, she got really bloated and sick. We knew then that she was intolerant to dairy and that it needed to be completely removed from her diet.

After two more weeks of the elimination diet, she had lost another 10 pounds. This time, however, we had eliminated wheat. When we reintroduced it back into her diet, she again got really sick, informing us that she also has sensitivity to wheat.

Overall, Julie lost a total of 21 pounds in four weeks. This is a normal outcome in our class, but she personally could not believe it. So she asked me, "The 21 pounds that I have lost—are those from fat?" My answer was no.

While Julie definitely lost some fat during that four-week period, it is nearly impossible for anyone to lose that much fat in such a short amount of time. Most of what Julie lost was unnecessary fluid manifesting itself as inflammation due to her diet consisting of various types of food that her body could not properly digest. Even so, I was much happier to remove her inflammation at that stage of her weight loss than I was to remove fat due to the fact that the excess inflammation was probably going to kill her. I know now that because she has less inflammation, her bowels are functioning better, her joint pain is minimized, and her chances of developing heart disease or cancer have decreased dramatically. She is happy that she has lost weight, but I am happy that she will be healthier.

I had another client join my weight-loss class that was morbidly overweight and suffering from a multitude of other health issues that were greatly interfering with her life. I instantly put her on an elimination diet, and within two weeks, she had lost 20 inches in her biographic dimensions and twelve pounds in weight. Moreover, to my delight, her lupus symptoms had been greatly reduced, and the red-blistered skin tainting her face had almost disappeared. I love to get such results!

Like so many others, this woman had come to me looking for weight loss, but what I ended up giving her was a healthier lifestyle, not just a thinner body. Unfortunately, in spite of her inspiring results, this client did not stick with my program, dropping out just shortly after she found herself improving. Other situations like this one have taught me a great deal in my experience with the program. Without going into too much detail, I think it would be beneficial to discuss some of those lessons here.

First, I have learned that I can't control people. Why would someone who is getting great results stop doing what is improving his or her overall health? It makes no sense to me. But I have learned that at the end of the day, people, including you, will do what they want—whether it makes sense to me or not.

Secondly, I have come to realize that some people are naturally destructive and do not want to get rid of their symptoms. Some feel that a disease can give them a badge of honor or a sense of identity. Hence, they feel that to lose their disease would be similar to discovering at thirty years old that they were adopted. Such a process can be utterly ego-shattering.

And thirdly, I have learned how to love people for who they are. I will try to help anyone who comes my way, but I cannot internalize or feel upset when a person does not follow through with my recommendations. People are free to do whatever they want. All I am required to do is to be there for them when they need me the most.

So it's up to you. Do you want to be healthy, or do you want to risk an early death by sticking to an unhealthy lifestyle? If you want to be healthy, then you might find it helpful to review and heed the following tips as you seek to give the elimination diet your best efforts.

Number one, in order to give yourself the best opportunity for success with the elimination diet, never plan to do an elimination diet close to Christmas, birthdays or family-get-togethers. It is difficult enough to do this special diet on a normal day, but you will find it doubly difficult when everyone around you is eating birthday cake. Therefore, plan to do the elimination diet during a time when you know that you won't have to entertain or eat whatever is placed in front of you. Set up your elimination diet phase for success by timing it properly. Don't set yourself up for failure by planning to perform your elimination diet over Christmas.

Secondly, in **Appendix B** you will find a questionnaire that will help you assess your food sensitivities. To begin, simply answer all of the questions and score all of your responses before you begin eliminating foods. Once you have completed three to four weeks of the elimination diet, go back and fill out the questionnaire again. Compare your resulting score with the score you attained three to four weeks ago. If your score has reduced dramatically through the elimination of certain foods, then you are most likely intolerant to those specific foods.

Thirdly, you need to constantly remind yourself that your belief that a certain food is healthy does not necessarily mean that it is healthy for you. Are cucumbers healthy? Yes, but not for me. I get bloated, irritable, and swollen to the point that I can't even take my wedding ring off. What dietician would state that cucumbers are not healthy? None of them. But I can tell you without a shadow of a doubt that they are not healthy for me. This dietary abnormality is a part of my individuality. It is how I was made. If I try to fight my genetic make-up and eat cucumbers, I will make myself sick.

One of the main purposes of performing an elimination diet is to give your body a quiet down-time during which you are not experiencing any ill side effects due to your previous diet. To ensure that your body receives this quiet time, you must be certain that you are eliminating everything that could possibly be causing symptoms while simultaneously staying on the diet long enough for your body to purge itself from those symptoms. In addition, along with those foods that commonly give people inflammation, you must attempt to be aware enough of your body to eliminate foods that you wouldn't normally suspect. If tomatoes sometimes give you acid reflux, you should eliminate them. If garlic has a tendency to reappear in your belches for 4-6 hours after you have eaten it, then consider it to be a possible suspect for food sensitivity. Because your genetics and intestinal integrity are unique to you, you can be sensitive to anything...not just the common food groups mentioned earlier. I have had patients with sensitivities to dairy, wheat, corn, eggs, alcohol, bananas and even chicken. I have learned that it can be anything.

To assist you in knowing which foods to eliminate, take a week or two before you start eliminating anything from your diet to think about everything you eat. Be on the lookout for foods that create excess gas, bloating, stomach pain, diarrhea, constipation, headaches or any such symptoms. Any food products that results in any of these symptoms must be eliminated from your diet during the elimination phase.

Maybe this confession will encourage you. I was introduced to the concept of food intolerances for the first time about 10 years ago. When I first heard about it, I highly doubted its validity. I had studied food allergies and was well aware of the negative effects foods can have on one's body if he or she is allergic to them. In fact, I even knew that my brother is highly allergic to beans—to the point that if he accidentally consumes even a small amount, his eyes and throat will swell shut in less than fifteen minutes. I knew that such symptoms were life-threatening and very real, but the fact was his condition could be discovered easily through a blood or skin-allergy test, taking all possibility of his reactions being psychosomatic out of the equation. I did not have to wonder if his condition was 'in his head' because there was a test to prove that it was not. That was the main reason I doubted the theory of food intolerances when I first heard about it.

It used to be that my thought processes were so deeply entrenched in the medical model of disease that if a formal test could not be administered to check for a suspected condition, then I believed that the existence of that condition was questionable at best. It wasn't for another two years that my test-based theory began to crack.

The crack started about eight years ago when my wife told me that she believed she was intolerant to wheat, a conclusion she had arrived at via the process of elimination. She claimed that after consuming certain foods containing wheat or its derivatives, she would feel bloated and irritable. Needless to say, I had a difficult time believing her. I had taken a vow that I would love her until the day we died, but who said that I had to believe everything she said?

Now, I do the majority of the cooking in our house, so in an attempt to catch her in the midst of false-thinking, I purposefully would sneak wheat into her diet. However, to my surprise, each time I would place wheat in her food, she could tell I had done so because she would suffer from excessive bloating. That's when I knew that there must be something to the theory of food intolerance.

Since that time, I have studied theories concerning food intolerances deeply and have experimented with the various theories with many of my patients. What I have learned has made me a committed believer. I know that many people unknowingly suffer from food intolerances and that their symptoms are numerous, severe and preventable.

I also know that food sensitivities rarely show up on allergy tests due to the nature of the tests and what they measure. Food allergies are determined by injecting a small amount of allergen (food particle) under a patient's skin and observing his or her skin's reaction. The reaction of a positive test is a reddening or rising of the skin at the site of the injection. Food sensitivities do not result in a positive reaction because it does not involve the immune system. For this reason, the topic of food sensitivities has been treated with suspicion by the medical community.

The term food intolerance is a general term that essentially denotes any food not tolerated well by an individual. It does not describe why that particular food is a problem in the first place. The most common and accepted way of describing why and how food intolerances occur in the human body is the one we explored above detailing milk and lactose intolerance. To be more specific this time, lactose is the sugar found in milk. People who are lactose intolerant suffer undesirable symptoms from the consumption of milk because they lack the enzyme lactase. This is a very necessary enzyme to digest milk. The lactose does not get broken down without it; leaving the normal bacteria cultures in your colon to feed upon its sugars. As a byproduct, the bacteria within your colon begin to produce large amounts of toxins and gas. This production of toxins accounts for any of the adverse effects (such as joint pain or headaches) you might experience after you drink the milk, while the excess gas production can account for any of the bloating or abdominal distension you may suffer.

The above example of intolerant digestion can be applied to any food product. If a person does not possess the necessary enzymes to properly digest a certain type of food, then symptoms similar to those accompanying lactose intolerance may arise.

There is another form of improper digestion that also might help to explain some of the food intolerances that you may be experiencing. This form of indigestion is known as intestinal permeability or leaky gut.

When healthy, your gastrointestinal tract creates a fortress between the digestion that is taking place within your intestines and your blood vascular system. However, research has shown that after an infection of influenza, excessive antibiotic usage, or chronic consumption of NSAID's (Aspirin, ibuprofens etc.), your barrier can break down, allowing the passage of foreign, undigested materials and pathogens into your bloodstream. Such a condition would make you appear to be sensitive to everything that you eat.

I have seen patients suffering from this form of indigestion in my office, and I will tell you that these people do not have food intolerances to any particular food but instead experience sensitivities to a broad variety of foods to the point that almost everything they eat makes them sick. In fact, they will tell you that they feel better when they eat nothing. But people have to eat in order to live. The problem is that as soon as these patients start eating again, their symptoms return because particles of their undigested food are leaking into their bloodstream. Not surprisingly, when they have allergy testing done, their results generally show allergic responses to dozens of foods.

The truth is that patients suffering from intestinal permeability will not improve until they repair their gut lining, thereby fixing their permeability problem. Once the integrity of their lining is restored, these patients can eat items that they once thought they were allergic to without suffering any symptoms.

Even though the above scenario does happen, I do not want you to understand traditional food intolerances in this way. Most patients who experience sensitivity to certain types of foods do not discover their sensitivity through a positive reading on an allergy test. Of course, some food sensitivities do cause allergic responses, but not all of them. If you do have an allergy test performed that indicates you are allergic to a food product, by all means, stay away from that food. But keep in mind that allergy tests will not necessarily indicate food sensitivities.

It is my opinion that the first scenario wherein a person does not have the proper enzymes to digest his or her food is a more common and likely explanation for food intolerances. You need specific enzymes to digest specific foods. We all know that we are unique on a genetic level. We understand that we possess unique genes that code for our unique characteristics, such as eye color and height. So why is it such a stretch to think that we also have different enzymes?

The best way to determine your perfect gene diet is via the process of the elimination diet. If you learn your specific dietary requirements through this process, I can state with confidence that you will prolong your life or, at the very least, experience less sickness.

Eat Rainbows

Our current knowledge of food and its importance has expanded tenfold in the past 50 years. What we thought we knew about how food is processed by the human body has taken a big detour. It used to be thought that food kept us alive, but now we know that it can also kill us by creating chronic inflammation and degenerative diseases. Understanding how American society's knowledge of food has changed over the years might make it easier to make wiser eating choices in the future.

During the Great Depression, many families were lucky to have any food on the table at mealtime and would not dare complain if it wasn't healthy for them. Today, we don't have the same threat, but our food industry has learned how to capitalize on our emotions with regards to this fear of food scarcity. I can still hear my grandmother and mother telling me to eat everything on my plate without griping, reminding me that there were starving people in Africa who would be lucky if they got any food at all.

This attitude of eat-it-and-don't-complain has permeated our society to the point that the unquestioning public has inadvertently given the food industry permission to add whatever they would like to food products as long as the additives prolong the food products' shelf lives. Hence, the food industry produces vast amounts of food products that no one would have even considered eating 80 years ago.

Nevertheless, Westernized countries have lost their sense of food scarcity and are beginning to question the sanity of unnecessary ingredients in their food. Why are so many additives being placed in our food? What are they doing to our health?

What we now know is that everything we do, eat, or drink causes oxidative stress. Please, don't get freaked out by that technical term. If the term oxidation scares you, just think of a cut apple, pear, or potato that turns brown very quickly after you cut it. That is oxidation. The problem is that oxidation can be the start of inflammation and once present in the body's tissues, very detrimental to your health. Thus, we need to eat foods that are antioxidants to prevent this from happening. Antioxidants are vitamins and plant extracts that go around binding up free radicals so they don't cause oxidation in you. The more of these foods that you eat, the less oxidative stress you will experience, and therefore the less inflammation. The less inflammation you have in your body's tissues, the less likely you will be to develop or perpetuate chronic and degenerative diseases. Simply put, if you will just keep in mind that antioxidant foods are also anti-inflammatory, you will be good to go. It's that simple.

"Without inflammation, it is pretty irrelevant what your cholesterol levels are."

Jonny Bowden and Stephen Sinatra authors of
The Great Cholesterol Myth

Our bodies are pretty good at dealing with short periods of inflammation, known as acute inflammation. However, long-term inflammation, or chronic inflammation, has a tendency to wear down the body to the point of permanent tissue damage. A good example of this is the way in which long-term inflammation in our arteries leads to atherosclerotic plaque (the hardening of our arteries), which can ultimately result in high blood pressure, a heart attack and eventually death.

Many types of cancer have been found to have the same root cause. Chronic, high levels of acid in your tissues may create chronic inflammation, tissue damage, and eventually cancer. In modern medicine, the treatment of choice has traditionally been to cut out the cancer or to shrink it with radiation or chemotherapy. This might be the prudent thing to do; however, this book has been written to focus on the prevention of disease. It is my hope that we can teach you to decrease your body's acid (oxidative stress) and thereby prevent the cancer from ever happening.

So where does food come into this picture? What does food have to do with causing inflammation, heart disease, diabetes, arthritis, and cancer? The answer is everything.

In short, your body creates free radicals when it digests and absorbs food. This is pretty much the same as saying that when your body digests and absorbs food; it is creating oxidative stress since free radicals are simply particles that bind to your tissues, causing the tissues to malfunction. It is this destruction of your tissues that creates chronic inflammation and begins the downward spiral towards cancer, heart disease, and many other diseases.

Some foods create more oxidative stress (free radicals) than others, and these are the foods that you should avoid. Some foods help prevent the binding of free radicals to your tissues, and these are the foods that you should eat more of. It is that simple.

Smoking and consuming excessive sodas will dramatically increase free radical and acid formation. Processed foods that are high in nitrates, preservatives, dyes, and artificial flavors have a tendency to create more free radicals. Foods that have a lot of natural color help prevent free radicals from binding to your tissues in the first place. For instance, the natural colors in green vegetables, red peppers, butternut squash, beets, blueberries, blackberries, and tomatoes all aid us in fighting oxidative stress. These foods neutralize acid and bind free radicals, successfully reducing chronic inflammation. Remember, by reducing chronic inflammation, you can dramatically reduce your chances of getting cancer or heart disease.

To make this concept easy for my son, ever since he was a little toddler, we have taught him to eat rainbows. In our family, that simply means that you have to eat food that has a lot of color. We make it a point to eat at least two to three colors each meal, and my son will tell you that the colors white or brown do not count. Why? Because the brighter the natural color in your food, the more effective it is in fighting inflammation. By consuming these foods you essentially prolong your life and help prevent cancer, diabetes, heart problems, and arthritis.

Moreover, each color of food has a separate and unique job. The blue pigments bind to certain free radicals, while the red ones bind to another, the greens yet to another. This is why your diet must be a rainbow consisting of all of the colors possibly found in food. To eat green beans with each meal is definitely better than not eating any color, but you are not preventing as much inflammation and as many diseases as compared to when you choose to eat a large variety of pigmented colors. This is one place in your life where more is better.

When I talk to patients about this concept, I invariably encounter those who complain that they don't like vegetables and therefore cannot follow my recommendation. I respond by telling them this. First of all, no one has to follow my recommendations. We live in a free country, and you don't have to listen to me. You are more than welcome to ignore my knowledge and die young. The choice is yours and only yours.

Secondly, who lied to you and made you believe that everything you put in your mouth must taste good? I never asked you if you like broccoli; I told you to eat it. You may not like colorful peppers, but who cares? Eat them anyway. Don't you know that the main function of food is to keep you alive and healthy? If you happen to also enjoy the food that is making you healthy, that is an extra bonus—not a prerequisite.

Eating good food, however, is a prerequisite, if you want to be healthy. If you are searching for love, purpose or belonging in food, you are headed down a dangerous path. The love you seek should be gotten from your family, friends, and life's purpose, not your food.

Nevertheless, I have had some patients try to eat healthy fruits and vegetables only to vomit. These patients are an enigma to me, so in an attempt to better understand them, I am slowly learning to experience life through their perspectives. The longer I practice, the more I understand. Thus, instead of asking them to continually make themselves ill, I give them the permission to take a whole-food supplement drink that will give them the antioxidants they need. To be sure, these supplements are not as good as getting all of their antioxidants from food, but they come very close. I will elaborate further on a great, whole-food supplement later in this book when I discuss vitamin supplementation.

Please note that I am not your personal doctor. I am well aware that many people have specific vitamin needs based on a particular disease or genetic problem. Therefore, before making radical changes in your diet, you should consult with your doctor. But be aware that many orthodox medical doctors do not believe food can directly affect your health or your sense of wellbeing. For this reason, if your doctor has a negative attitude towards diet modifications, please become educated and make your own diet decisions. However, if your personal doctor is well-versed in dietary needs, be sure to listen to his or her recommendations.

To start eating in rainbows, see **Appendix A** for a sample list of foods that you should eat and a list of those that you should avoid. Keep in mind that foods you are intolerant of should be avoided at all costs, even if you see those foods on the list of "thing to eat." Like I said earlier, removing foods you are intolerant towards is probably one of the most important things you can do for your health. What might be healthy for one person may not necessarily be healthy for you.

Often patients ask me which particular foods treat different types of conditions or symptoms. However, I have purposefully omitted that topic from this book for several reasons. Foremost, I want my patients to be eating a variety of healthy foods, not just one particular kind because they have high cholesterol or acid reflux. When a person eats the types of foods listed in Appendix A, they will be fighting every condition possible that is due to diet.

Secondly, I do not want to advocate the theory that food should be treated as medicine. The average person is so entrenched in the traditional medical model that he or she assumes specific foods fight specific conditions. This presupposes that food is nothing more than a collection of vitamins and nutrients and that those particular vitamins fight particular conditions. The problem with this theory of reductionism is that it removes the vital properties of food. Food is greater than the sum of all its parts. If it were not, we could eat pills alone and attain everything we need to survive. You and I both know that is not the case.

Lesson 1: Diet is the most important factor in living healthily and preventing diseases.

Points to Remember

1. Eat foods that are less processed and do not contain artificial food additives, flavor enhancers, dyes, preservatives or chemical additives. Foods consisting of these harmful ingredients cannot be broken down properly by your digestive tract and may result in chronic inflammation resulting in disease.

2. Start the process of an elimination diet to determine your unique food intolerances. By removing foods that you cannot digest, you will reduce inflammation and more effectively maintain your weight. Remember that what is healthy for one person may cause inflammation for the next. By removing food intolerances, you dramatically reduce your chances of getting sick.

3. Eat all of the colors of the rainbow. Each color you consume will help you fight off free radicals, reduce acid and in doing so, will help you to reduce inflammation. Reducing inflammation will help you minimize your chances of developing the common inflammatory diseases such as heart disease, arthritis, diabetes and even cancer

"Water is the most neglected nutrient in your diet but one of the most vital."

Kelly Barton

Lesson 2

Water: Not Just for the Fishes

According to Wikipedia, the human body consists of anywhere between 60-75% water. How is it possible that generally we don't even like something so basic to our make-up and so necessary for our survival? We have grown up in the Coke-or-Pepsi generation for so long that a big glass of cold water just doesn't seem that appealing anymore. All the while, high fructose corn syrup, phosphoric acid, and artificial colors simply increase our bodies' toxic loads and lead us blindly towards obesity and disease.

Nevertheless, I am not an extremist. I would never claim that you should never drink a carbonated soda. I wouldn't even claim that I haven't partaken in a cold Pepsi from time to time. However, the majority of our population does not indulge in soda as just a treat. They rely on it as their sole form of liquid. I regularly have patients tell me that they have anywhere from six to eight cans of soda a day…yet they wonder why they are sick.

Now I will admit, there are very few things as good as going to a movie and snacking on a large popcorn while sipping on a large soda. But for me, that is a lavish treat, not an everyday occurrence.

Water has been called the universal solvent. This means that water is needed to perform most of the biochemical reactions that take place in your body. Without proper hydration, your body cannot function properly, and you will end up feeling sick. Your muscles cannot contract without proper hydration. Your brain cannot think without water, and most importantly of all for this book, your body cannot lose excess fat properly without adequate amounts of water. According to Dr. Batmanghelidj, who is an expert on water and the author of the book *Your Body's Many Cries for Water*, water can also be used to treat the symptoms of ulcers, migraines and high blood pressure. This is because dehydration can cause excessive constriction in your blood vessels, which is very often the trigger for high blood pressure and migraines. Since this is the case, starting a daily regiment of consuming cold water throughout the day could both improve your dehydration as well as cool down your body temperature, which could ultimately prevent migraines. In addition, rehydrating your blood vessels will cause them to dilate, thereby reducing your blood pressure.

In my weight-loss class, I have seen many patients lose as much as 10 pounds simply by drinking more water. I am passionate about teaching my patients this easy concept because I know the importance of water and how dramatically it can improve their lives. For this reason, when it comes to levels of importance, I believe that water consumption is the second most important factor in living longer and healthier.

Often when I introduce the topic of water consumption to my patients, I get asked questions about the additives and foreign substances that are now found in our drinking water. Surely we have all heard about the chemicals that can be found in our drinking water, especially since the Internet practically overflows with information regarding the bad effects of water-born molecules. One source will tell you to only drink bottled water, while another claims that tap water is just as good. So who should you believe?

If you are like many of my patients, you don't have the time or resources to research everything that goes into your body.

Unfortunately, this makes it easier for you to be led astray by propaganda often presented by random organizations that build their profits off of human ignorance. Aware of this, it is my hope that this book will clarify some of your potential questions.

Most bottled waters prove more pure than tap water. However, we now know that the plastic bottles used by bottling companies contain a toxic chemical known as bisphenol A or BPA. When this chemical finds its way into the human body, it acts similarly to the body's natural hormone estrogen. Environmental chemicals that act similar to estrogen are called xenoestrogens.

Consuming external sources of estrogen, such as the xenoestrogens found in plastic bottles, may result in abnormally high levels of estrogen. If perpetuated, this can lead to estrogen-based cancers such as breast or uterine cancer. One of the most rapidly growing cancers in men today is breast cancer, which could be due to their excessive consumption of xenoestrogens.

In comparison, tap water is filtered from a local reservoir and then purged of its bacteria, viruses, and protozoans through the addition of chlorine. This is a great thing to do except for the fact that the filtration methods used do not filter many toxic substances. In one study that FoxNews.com reported, dangerous quantities of prescription drugs were found in the water of 24 American cities. In addition, despite the fact that chlorine is necessary in our water to kill off dangerous parasites, it may also cause harm to the human body if consumed in large quantities.

The question remains: What is the best form of water to drink? Let's answer that question by taking a look at what I do for my family. I have placed a filtration system under my sink that removes chlorine and other unwanted substances from my drinking water. I use this filtered water for everything—drinking, cleaning fruits and vegetables and also cooking. I choose to do this for two reasons. First and foremost, it saves me money when compared to buying bottled water containing harmful BPA. And secondly, it ensures that the food I cook does not contain the toxins and chlorine I am so diligently trying to avoid in my drinking water. To put it another way, it makes absolutely no sense in my mind for me to avoid drinking toxic-free water if I am still going to boil pasta and wash my veggies with polluted water, especially since using the filtration system takes no more effort than using regular tap water once it is hooked up.

Moreover, to ensure that no BPA sneaks into my filtered water when I go to drink it, I make sure that I pour my filtered water into a BPA-free, plastic container or glass. Without this precaution, it is pointless to have the filtration system in the first place since I would likely be consuming BPAs from my plastic bottle anyway.

You too can avoid the dangerous toxins found in plastic bottles and tap water by purchasing and installing a filtration system under your sink from your local hardware store. The one I currently have under my kitchen sink cost approximately $50 and only needs to be replaced every six months. This is a cheap price to pay when it comes to living healthily and preventing diseases.

Learning to drink clean water should raise another question: How much clean water should a healthy person drink?

I generally use a calculation in my weight-loss program that stands upon the assumption that a 200-pound person needs to drink more water than a 100-pound person. In other words, this calculation states that you should consume half of your body weight in ounces every day. That means that if you weigh 200 pounds, you need to consume one hundred ounces of water each day. If you weigh 100 pounds, you should consume fifty ounces of water a day.

Rarely do I have a patient who consumes that much water, but the closer you get to that value the better. Keep in mind that fresh fruits and vegetables hold a lot of water and add greatly to your recommended intake of water each day.

Fruit juices also count towards your daily intake of water, but be aware that the fiber naturally found in the fruit from which the juice is made has been removed during the juicing process. This makes the sugars in the juice highly absorbable, which can cause your body to struggle with regulating its blood sugar concentration. Consumed often enough, high amounts of absorbed sugar can induce conditions such as hyperglycemia (high blood sugar) and will increase your chances of diabetes and obesity. Fruit juices are not evil, but consume them in moderation. The best fluid is and always will be clean water.

Drinks that do not count towards your daily water intake include caffeinated drinks such as sodas, teas, and coffee. In contrast, these drinks can actually be detrimental to your body by causing water loss. This is because the caffeine in these drinks is a diuretic, which is a fancy way of saying that these products make you pee out more fluid than you consume, causing dehydration. Now, I am not telling you that you can never drink caffeinated beverages. I am simply going to advise you how I counsel my patients: If you consume eight ounces of caffeinated coffee, tea, or whatever, you must offset the dehydrating effect of the caffeine on your body by consuming an additional eight ounces of non-caffeinated fluid. Like I said, caffeinated beverages are not forbidden, but you will need to consume more fluids to compensate for their ill effects.

All of your body's cellular processes that are fueled by water are still capable of working if you are dehydrated, but they will do so with less effectiveness. In some situations, the processes will be slowed down, and in other instances, the processes will be sped up. Either way, you can be sure that if your cells are dehydrated, you cannot operate at your peak. Your muscles and brain will function at a slower rate. You will not be able to repair your cells and tissues as fast. And you will age more rapidly and show more wrinkles. Simply put...most people are dehydrated and should drink more water. Not many things in life are so simple, so cheap and still so effective. So why stay dehydrated?

Just Say No to the Halides: Chlorine, Bromine, and Fluoride

Many of my patients have trouble losing weight. They have tried many diet programs only to fail and become more frustrated. Admittedly, there can be many reasons for their failure. There is one factor that I would like to talk about here that may not only help you lose weight, but might also make you healthier. The name of this factor is hypothyroidism.

Hypothyroidism occurs when your thyroid gland (which is located in your neck, just in front of your windpipe) is not functioning properly due to not secreting enough thyroid hormone. The lower secretions of this gland will dramatically reduce your metabolism and result in weight gain, chronic fatigue and even depression. Your doctor will generally prescribe Synthroid or Armour to help you regulate your body's thyroid metabolism and in turn, your weight management and energy levels. This method, though necessary, is rarely effective. I will explain why.

As a rule, a thyroid gland that is functioning normally does not have a constant level of secretions. Instead, the normal thyroid gland will secrete low amounts of thyroid hormone when it is time for the body to sleep and higher amounts of hormone when it is time for the body to be awake. These natural fluctuations of thyroid hormone render medicine's attempt to maintain a consistent blood level of thyroid hormone ineffective. Not only that, but secretions of thyroid hormone that do not ebb and flow with the rhythms of daily life can make a person feel like a zombie with too much energy to sleep but not enough energy to function properly. Patients suffering from such problems generally become morbidly obese and extremely frustrated due to their inability to lose weight despite their attempts to consume less food. With these facts in mind, I will illustrate how we can help manage this dysfunction while simultaneously following principles for anyone who wishes to stay healthy.

The hormone that the thyroid gland secretes, thyroxin, requires iodine. There are several chemicals that are similar to iodine on a molecular level. When a person has been exposed to these elements in large amounts, his or her thyroid can kick out the needed iodine from the gland and leave the patient experiencing the symptoms of hypothyroidism. In this case, the body is producing thyroid hormone, but the hormone is being rendered ineffective. Chemicals that provoke this self-defeating behavior in the thyroid are **chlorine**, **bromine**, and **fluoride**. These three chemicals make up a family of elements called the halides.

Fluoride is found in your toothpaste and is used to kill bacteria in your mouth. Bromine gets put in your hot tubs to kill bacteria in the hot water. Chlorine resides in your swimming pools and tap water to kill bacteria in drinking water. It is obvious from the list I just gave you that these chemicals, including iodine, are used to kill pathogens such as bacteria and viruses within water. Hence, chlorine is very necessary if you want clean drinking water to be delivered to your home. The point is that once clean water has been delivered, it is not necessary to consume the added chlorine that aided in the filtration process. In fact, a person who is exposed to large amounts of halide chemicals, such as chlorine, may be unintentionally setting themselves up or perpetuating thyroid dysfunction and excessive weight gain.

Below I have listed the counsel I give my patients who suffer from thyroid dysfunction. Throughout this process, my goal is always to repair their thyroid glands and to improve their health. I never seek to remove a patient from the medication that has been prescribed by his or her doctor. However, you will find that more progressive doctors will reduce or eliminate a patient's medication once their dysfunction is repaired.

First, it is important to immediately remove all of your exposure to chlorine, bromine, and fluoride. While this may sound daunting, the elimination can be as simple as buying non-fluoride toothpaste. Such toothpastes may be a little more expensive and slightly harder to find, but your local health food store should keep such toothpastes on their shelves. As with other things, if there are a variety of non-fluoride toothpastes from which to choose, you need to buy the one containing the least amount of added chemicals.

Secondly, if you are using bromine in a hot tub, you need to begin using an alternative. I personally use a silver stick that has been long-known to kill bacteria. These are easy to install, and your local pool supply store should have them in stock. Though I do have to keep my hot tub pump running more frequently as well as clean the filters more often, the potential gains far outweigh the extra work.

Lastly, you must remove chlorine from your life. In fact, I would contend that this is the most important part of the equation when you are trying to repair a low-functioning thyroid. As mentioned earlier, you must never drink or cook with chlorinated water. You can avoid doing so by putting a filter on your cold-water tap in your kitchen. This will prevent chlorine from slipping into your coffee, water glass, and cooked or washed food.

Along the same lines, you must also place a filter on your shower head to inhibit chlorine from being absorbed into your skin or your lungs. Both the skin and the lining of your lungs are the largest surface areas in your body. If you don't eliminate the exposure of your lungs and skin to chlorine, it is highly unlikely that you will be able to reduce enough exposure in your drinking water to have any appreciable effect.

I mentioned previously that I purchased a filter for my kitchen sink for about $50. You can buy a filter for your shower for approximately $25. Moreover, filters for your shower head can be installed easily by simply unscrewing your shower head, attaching the filter, and reattaching the shower head. The whole process takes less than five minutes and only has to be repeated for replacement once a year. These are small prices to pay for clean water that may prevent you from developing hypothyroidism.

For obvious reasons, swimming pools are one of the hardest water sources to control when it comes to chlorine exposure. Whether you own your own swimming pool or you use one at your local gym, it is impossible to swim in a clean pool without chlorine. For that reason, I warn any patient that I am assisting in repairing hypothyroidism to stay away from swimming pools. Once they have been cured from this affliction, they might be able to have chlorine exposure in limited amounts such as going to the pool occasionally. However, when you are in the process of repairing your thyroid gland, you must avoid swimming pools at all costs.

After you eliminate your body's exposure to chlorine, bromine, and fluoride you may then start vitamin supplementation with iodine to excessively load the body with iodine so that it can enter the thyroid gland and repair the damage. This process of repair may take several months, but it generally works well.

Please note that even if you don't have a thyroid dysfunction, the above method can be used to prevent hypothyroidism and keep your metabolism highly functional. You may not have to supplement your diet with iodine, but the removal of the excessive chlorine, bromine, and fluoride can still be useful in the prevention of diseases.

Lesson 2: Drink more water.

Points to Remember

1. Water is one of the most necessary and beneficial substances on the planet. Many diseases can be cured and prevented by drinking more water.

2. Liquid beverages other than water, such as sodas, coffee, alcohol and sports drinks are not substitutes for clean, pure water. If you drink caffeinated beverages, you must drink additional non-caffeinated fluids to compensate for the dehydrating effects of caffeine.

3. Each person should drink half of their body weight in ounces every day. For example, if you weigh 200 pounds, you need to consume one hundred ounces of water each day.

4. Store your water in BPA-free containers to prevent excessive exposure to estrogen-like compounds found in plastics.

5. Install a filter on your kitchen faucet to get clean drinking and cooking water. Also, install a filter on your shower head to remove excessive exposure to chlorine from your skin and lungs.

"It's paradoxical that the idea of living a long life appeals to everyone, but the idea of getting old doesn't appeal to any one."

Andy Rooney

Lesson 3

Exercise:
How Much Is Too Much?

In the not-so-distant past, most people had physical jobs that made the thought of extra physical exercise as foreign as speaking Urdu. However, most people today have desk jobs that demand little to no activity. And not only that, but by the time most people return home at the end of the day, they feel exhausted and too drained to do any exercise. This lack of physical activity combined with the fact that our lives are extremely stressful significantly contributes to our natural distaste for exercise.

Exercise is one of the most important things that you can do for your health. Proper exercise can increase your lean muscle mass, improve your body's hormone production, reduce signs of aging, improve your moods, strengthen your bone density, and even help in preventing heart disease. If exercise were a pill, people would be popping it like crazy. But it is not that simple, is it? Instead, we all have to get off of our comfortable chairs and find the mental fortitude to exercise.

Now more than ever, we need physical activity in our daily routines, especially since it can be a great stress reducer, help with weight management, prevent certain diseases, and improve energy and overall vitality. But when I speak to patients about exercise, I invariably get the deer-caught-in-the-headlights blank stare telling me that they either don't want to exercise or that they don't know which exercises to do. It never fails, though, that once they hear what I have to say, they become much more receptive.

You see, the majority of my patients equate exercising with running marathons or trying to keep up with Richard Simmons "Sweating to the Oldies." But as one of my wise professors once told me, "The best exercise for a patient is any exercise that patient will do." And I can tell you that, by and large, my patients do not like to do excessive exercising. Hence, if I told one of them to start jogging, you can be sure that he or she would not do it. However, excessive exercise is not something I write down on my patients' treatment plans. In fact, not only do I not promote excessive exercise, I also believe that intense exercise can be detrimental to people's health, possibly leading to arthritis and chronic disease. Let me explain.

In our first lesson, we talked about how every process of life creates oxidative stress, free radicals, and high acid in the human body. We spoke about how smoking and consuming excessive sodas may increase acid and start a disease process in your body. It may come as a shock for you to learn, then, that exercise also creates excessive acid and oxidative stress in the human body. Thus, in many instances, exercise actually can be considered dangerous and detrimental to your health because it dramatically increases so many toxic substances in your body. These toxins can lead to chronic inflammation, heart disease, and possibly cancer.

Let's think about this for a minute. I'm sure you have known people who were the perfect picture of fitness and health. They jogged every day, ran marathons, and looked great. Yet they died in their fifties. I'm sure you also know excessively obese people who look horrible but continue to live well into their eighties. Does body composition really determine your quality of life or even your life span? To make it simple, I have this saying, "If you are not going to eat right, I'd rather you be a couch potato."

What I'm essentially getting at is, because excessive exercise increases blood acid levels and oxidative stress, you must have a diet high in antioxidants, found in rainbow color foods, to counteract those detrimental effects. If you don't eat a diet high in antioxidants, then you had better exercise very little in life. Otherwise, you will only be increasing your blood acid and oxidative stress to the point that you will get sick and die prematurely.

Many thin people think that because they are thin they can eat whatever they want. Indeed, some thin people only eat deep-fried foods with little to no fruits and vegetables and don't drink enough water every day yet still don't gain weight. These individuals may look healthy on the outside, but I'm telling you that their lifestyle will kill them regardless of whether they are fat or thin.

So what is the answer? On the surface, it seems like whether you exercise or not you will die...but not necessarily.

Physical activity is important. Increasing your heart rate and moving your body can prevent heart disease, reduce obesity, and minimize arthritic pain. But excessive exercise can be detrimental. I personally believe that you should not exercise more than 20 to 30 minutes on any given day. Exercising more than that will increase your body's formation of acid as well as cause it to produce too much cortisol, a hormone not only linked to excessive feelings of stress, but also to the breakdown of much needed body muscle.

Also, if you are going to exercise, even at this reduced level of 20 to 30 minutes several days a week, you must compensate for your body's acid formation by consuming high antioxidant foods such as fruits, berries, and colorful vegetables. Myself, I consume an antioxidant shake within moments after I exercise to negate the ill effects of oxidation that my exercise produced. I will discuss this shake product in the chapter on vitamin supplementation; however, please note that I am not a proponent of excessive vitamin use. Consumption of vitamins in pill form should only be done when a person does not consume enough healthy foods, which I am also sometimes guilty of.

So, if you're going to exercise, which types of exercise should you do? Opinions on this greatly differ, I will tell you what I believe. There are many people who would argue with valid points on this subject. Nevertheless, I am going to present you with what I believe is the golden standard of exercise for any person who wants to live a healthy life that is composed of proper weight management and disease prevention.

If you observe the animal kingdom, you will notice that most animals classified as long-distance runners have four legs. Animals with two legs generally don't run long distances. For instance, have you ever seen an ape or a chicken running a 26-mile marathon? Humans have two legs. We are not built for long-distance running. The human race was built for strength, and quick bursts of energy. Forcing our bodies to do things that they were not meant to do can result in bodily dysfunction and diseases. I can't tell you how many patients have come into my office looking for help with knee pain and hip pain from running or biking. These activities are brutal on your joints and should be done sparingly.

To best describe the types of exercises I think are healthy, it is best that I give you my routine. I exercise 25 to 30 minutes two or three times a week. Two of those days generally consist of weight lifting during which I focus on my upper body one day and my lower body the next. If I decide to exercise on the third day, I spend about 20 to 30 minutes of moderate aerobic exercise on an elliptical machine. I personally choose an elliptical machine because it is less detrimental to my knee joints than other aerobic exercises.

In regards to weight lifting, I pay close attention to balance. If I weight lift using the muscles in the front of my arms, then I follow up that exercise with lifting weights using the muscles in the back of my arms. Likewise, if I lift with my chest muscle, I follow up those repetitions with a back exercise. When I lifted with the front of my legs, I also do an exercise that stresses the back of my legs. Balance in your exercise routine will prevent many chronic injuries while also maintain neurological health— a point that we will dig deeper into when we discuss the importance of chiropractic care.

So why do I exercise the way that I do? First of all, most people have a wrong understanding about why they should exercise. Weight management gurus have always told us that the key to weight loss is to consume less food calories while exercising more to burn all of our excess calories. If that were true, wouldn't you see more thin people in gyms? After all, we've been cutting our calories and working out more for decades, and our nation is fatter now than it has ever been. Have you ever noticed that you can run on a treadmill while its computer counts the amount of calories you have burned? The average person can run relatively fast on a treadmill for about 45 minutes to one hour and only burn 100-150 calories. That is less calories than one piece of chicken. At that rate, you would have to live on the treadmill to burn enough calories to negate your daily intake of food. It is ridiculous.

There are several reasons to exercise, and calorie burning is way down on the list. If you do a stretching routine, you will increase your flexibility and range of motion, but you will not build muscle or increase your heart and lung function. If you do any form of aerobic exercise, you will dramatically improve your heart and lung function but have very little gains on muscle growth and hormone stimulation. If you choose to do an anaerobic exercise, such as weight lifting, your heart and lung function will improve some, but the main gains would be in your muscle growth and hormone production.

With these things in mind then, the exercise that you choose to do should be based on the outcome you wish to have. If you are concerned with heart disease due to having already had a heart attack or because heart trouble runs in your family, it would be prudent to do some aerobic (cardiovascular) exercise. If you have chronic stiffness and limited joint mobility, as is common with arthritis, then stretching would be a better choice. But if you have stepped foot in a gym, you will notice most people exercise to maintain or lose weight.

I personally teach a weight-loss class with which I have had tremendous results and success. My weight-loss program has many different facets, some of which are covered in this book. But with regards to exercise, I teach that the best way to lose fat weight and keep it off is to gain muscle strength and muscle volume. The best exercise to accomplish that goal is—you guessed it—weight lifting.

Weight lifting is, by far, the best way to gain muscle volume and stimulate proper hormone function. As Jamie Jamieson and Dr. L. E. Dorman so eloquently attest in their book *Growth Hormone: Reversing Human Aging Naturally*, weight lifting has been proven to stimulate testosterone and human growth hormone. They assert that heavy weight lifting is one of the best ways to stimulate growth hormone production and reverse the signs of aging.

That is why I use heavy weights when I lift. I make sure that the weights are heavy enough that I can only do six to eight repetitions with them, but light enough that I can still maintain proper form while doing those repetitions. The intensity of this workout causes my muscles to grow faster, increases my hormone production and builds my strength. All of these aspects have been known to slow aging, increase vitality, and decrease a person's chances for developing diabetes or becoming obese.

This is a great time to remind you of a point that I made earlier. Exercise creates oxidative stress and increases your acid production. Hence, you must consume plenty of antioxidant foods to negate this problem. I personally drink a vitamin supplement called Greens First right after I exercise. One serving of this product is equivalent to the antioxidant capacity of 15 servings of vegetables. I also consume about 25 grams of protein within twenty minutes of finishing my workout to give my body the necessary building blocks for creating more muscle. Instead of drinking a high protein shake, you could also eat protein in the form of a meat product.

In the book *The Cortisol Connection*, Dr. Shawn Talbott reports that lifting weights intensely for short durations of time will reduce your chances of stimulating cortisol. Cortisol is a necessary but nasty hormone for anyone wanting to lose excess body weight because it often breaks down their muscle mass, which is detrimental to keeping off weight.

Therefore, because of the adverse effects of cortisol, if I have a patient or client who insists on running on a treadmill for more than 20 minutes, I make sure that he or she is doing so at a moderate pace. That is, the pace of their running is not inhibiting them from carrying on a conversation. I also insist that these patients perform the exercise with their eyes closed, if possible, and picture a tranquil scene that relaxes them. This will reduce the stress perceived by their bodies and reduce their cortisol production.

Bearing all of these things in mind then, I think we can begin to see why many weight-loss programs fail. Most programs are only interested in a person losing weight and generally pay little attention to helping their client's gain muscle. In my weight-loss classes, I use a computer device to calculate how much muscle and how much fat a person has. Our goal is to reduce the fat percentage while increasing the muscle percentage. The overall effect will be fat loss without the nasty burden of gaining it back over time.

I exercise this way because I have no yearning to become obese as I age or to look as if I am rapidly aging. My goal is to die very old and in great shape. So, exercise to keep your body fit and healthy, but don't exercise excessively so as to increase your chances of getting a disease or dying young. Also remember, anyone who exercises must have a better diet than non-exercising people to counteract the acid that exercise causes.

Lesson 3: Exercise.

Points to Remember

1. Exercise two or three times a week for a maximum of 25-30 minutes.

2. Excessive exercise can cause problems and may even shorten your life expectancy.

3. Choose the appropriate exercise for your desired outcome. Stretch for flexibility. Do aerobic exercises for improving your heart and lung function. And lift weights to increase your muscle volume and aid in weight management.

4. Weight lifting should be done with heavy weights and low repetitions to get maximum gains.

5. Consume a high antioxidant drink or eat plenty of fruits and vegetables to counteract the negative effects of exercise.

"Healthy citizens are the greatest asset any country can have."

Winston S. Churchill

Lesson 4

Chiropractic Is a Must: Move Your Bones Now, or You Won't Move Them Later

Chiropractic manipulation has two major effects on the human body. One: it improves joint movement. Two: it improves neurological function. Because this profession has been greatly misunderstood, I will attempt to illustrate why every person walking the planet needs to be adjusted by a chiropractor from time to time...whether he or she is in pain or not.

I have heard it said that nothing is really alive unless it moves. A stone can hardly be classified as living since it has no capacity to stand up or move locations by itself. Living things move, grow and procreate. When human beings were created, they were designed with joints and muscles to aid them in this much-needed motion. You have a joint in your arm because your elbows were meant to move. You do not have a joint in the middle of your forearms because you were not meant to move there. It is that simple.

As we observed in the previous lesson, modern life has become very lethargic. Most people have desk jobs prohibiting them from moving their joints enough to keep them healthy. Let me explain.

Every place where two bones meet in your body is a joint. As a rule, because joints don't have a very good blood supply, oxygen and nutrition can only get into them via motion. Likewise, waste products, such as lactic acid, can't get out of our joints unless we move them. Body tissues that have a more adequate blood supply can get oxygen and nutrients to the tissues and remove waste products simply by the beating of your heart. But joints are not so lucky. For joints, no movement or abnormal movement means no circulation of fluids, this leads to degeneration, a painful condition called arthritis. Once a joint becomes arthritic, it produces a lot of inflammation that can spread throughout the body causing diseased tissue elsewhere.

So simply put, a joint that moves properly and often is a healthy joint free of arthritis. Yoga, palates, or general stretching can help you keep your joints moving and healthy. Walking may also help to prevent arthritis in your feet, knees, and hips, but be aware that merely walking will achieve little movement in your spine.

For the reasons stated above, chiropractors use joint manipulation to get locked joints moving. For instance, let's assume that you are bending forward to touch your toes. Encasing the lower part of your spinal cord, you have five lumbar vertebrae that should each bend a little to give you full range of motion assuming your joints are healthy. However, if you bend forward and only four of your five vertebrae move, then you have one vertebra that is locked. This locking or lack of motion will result in improper fluid circulation within the joints of that vertebra and thus start the degenerative, arthritis process. Also, because you are now forcing the unlocked vertebrae to move more to compensate for the one that is stuck, those too will experience damage due to excessive motion.

Any bone that experiences improper motion will become arthritic first, but the other neighboring joints will soon follow. Just as a seed will grow and spread, so also will arthritis in your joints. I have been a chiropractor for over a decade, and I can't tell you how many patients I have X-rayed only to find severe arthritis spreading from their lower backs into the middle of their backs and necks. Sadly, if those patients would have just chosen to have their spine adjusted periodically, the original joint that was damaged would have been found and corrected before the inflammation spread, sparing those patients the agony of full-spine arthritis.

Chiropractors are highly skilled at finding locked vertebrae and getting them to move properly while concurrently leaving the fully functional joints alone. By having your spine adjusted, all of your joints will move properly and thereby decrease your chances for arthritis.

Great chiropractors can also unlock joints that are not spinal, such as your wrists, feet, elbows, and knees. As with your spinal joints, unlocking these joints can prevent joint dysfunction and arthritis from developing. The problem is that many times you are not going to be able to tell when a joint is locked because the pain or lack of mobility that often informs you of a locked joint is not present. For this reason, monthly check-ups are a must if you want to live a healthy life.

I currently have hundreds of patients who come into my office for a check-up once a month. They truly understand what we are trying to accomplish. They know that they can't determine when they need an adjustment, and they fully embrace the truth that an ounce of prevention is worth a pound of cure.

The second and probably the most important function of a chiropractic adjustment is the act of balancing your nervous system. There are two main ways that an adjustment can affect your nervous system. Admittedly, the explanations for these effects can get really complicated, so I will attempt to keep it as simple as possible to give you an understanding of this concept.

Let's start by taking a brief look at the nervous system. In short, your brain is like your body's master computer. It controls everything that happens within your body, allowing you to move and feel things happening around and within your body. It also has many functions that you cannot feel, like regulating your heart beat, controlling the dilation and constriction of your blood vessels, as well as regulating your liver, pancreas, digestion of food, and a million other processes too numerous to mention.

The brain communicates with these millions of tissues mainly through your spinal cord. In that way, your spinal cord serves as the operator that sends your brain's communications to the rest of your body. This makes your spinal cord and its associated spinal nerves so important that it has to be encased in a shell of hard bone for protection, otherwise known as the vertebral column. If your spinal column had no joints, it would be protected even better, but you would move as though you were made from wood. The spinal joints allow your body to bend and move in all sorts of contortions, ultimately giving you the freedom to function better.

Hence, not only can fixations and misalignments of the spinal bones cause arthritis, they also can interfere with your brain's communication to the rest of your body by inhibiting the line of communication that travels from your brain to your tissues on the other end of your spine. This decrease in communication to the body can result in many different problems. For instance, I have had many patients with high blood pressure due to their spines being misaligned. Once fixed, their blood pressure improved. As a chiropractor, I am not directly trying to lower my patients' blood pressure, but it is the case that I am trying to fix their spines. And one of the beneficial side effects of fixing a person's spine is lowered blood pressure. Finally! A side effect that improves the way you feel without making things worse.

Another example of the way chiropractic adjustment can positively affect your body is this: whether you realize it or not, your body is constantly healing itself. Generally, without realizing, you are constantly injuring tissues, blood vessels, skin and nerves on all levels within your body. Healing doesn't stop when you sleep, eat, exercise, or play with your kids. No, your body's efforts to heal itself are controlled by your brain and central nervous system through their communication with the cells of your body via the nerves that exit from your spine. Chiropractic adjustments work with these nerves to aid in proper communication. In that way, chiropractic care improves and regulates healing.

Because of this natural, healing process, if your chiropractor finds areas in your spine that are not moving correctly, it is important to fix those damaged areas. Otherwise, the nerves travelling to that area will be suppressed. Many people think that chiropractic adjustments are only about managing pain, but that is just a glorious side effect of what chiropractors actually do.

The second way chiropractic care affects the nervous system is a bit more complicated, but I'm sure you will understand the basic premise.

Just as the brain is always sending messages to your body's tissues, it is also constantly getting information from your body's tissues. Mostly we just think about the feelings of touch, heat, pressure, vibration and other sensations, but did you know that your brain also gets messages with regard to how your heart, liver, and other organs feel? For simplicity's sake, I will talk about sensation, communications from your body.

Let's say that your brain is receiving information from a vertebra in your lower spine. The nerves communicating that message are located on the left, right, front and back of your lower vertebra. If the sensations being communicated on the left and right side of your vertebra are equal, then your brain will determine that everything is working great. But if, say, the nerves on the left side of your vertebra report more sensation than the nerves on the right, your brain will determine that there is something wrong, letting you know that there is an imbalance by giving you the sense that you are dizzy or that your muscles are tight due to getting less sensation. When this tightness happens in your back, it can bring pain with it.

Therefore, vertebrae that do not move correctly almost always have nerves that are firing unequally, causing an imbalance of sensation that normally results in dizziness or muscle spasms in the imbalanced area. Your body wants to be balanced; thus it will always function better when it is.

Chiropractors are trained to balance and regulate the nervous system, allowing your body to know where your damaged tissues are so that it can initiate the healing process. Hence, there is no person on this planet who cannot benefit from a chiropractic adjustment. We all have spines, and we all have nerves attached to our spines that communicate with our bodies. Thereby, we all need adjustments.

As you can hopefully now see: there are many symptoms that can improve and even vanish after chiropractic treatment. However, the chiropractic adjustment was not designed to cure anything. The adjustment was only meant to reduce the interference of the nervous system at the spinal level. Once a nerve is allowed to operate undisturbed, the function of that nerve returns to its normal activity, including the activity of healing the tissues that it connects. I hope that this explanation enables you to see that your chiropractor does not heal you. It is your body that heals you. Your chiropractor simply sets the stage that allows your body to function properly enough to heal itself.

Generally, patients come to a chiropractor for spinal pain, and as a result of having an adjustment, their spinal pain is reduced. However, because the real goal of chiropractic care is to restore nerve function in the body so that it can resume its proper activity, it is not uncommon to see a variety of conditions within patients improve. Throughout my years of practice, I have seen countless patients with a variety of conditions get better. I have seen patients previously unable to have children get pregnant, and others suffering from stomach pain find relief. I have seen patients with diabetes get to the point that they only need a fraction of the insulin they previously relied upon, while the emotional disorders of depression, anxiety, and suicidal tendencies have vanished in others. I have witnessed children with symptoms of attention deficit disorder dramatically improve, as well as a number of other symptoms go away.

Now please understand, I am not suggesting that if you have a terminal illness or chronic condition that you should abandon traditional treatment and only see a chiropractor. What I am suggesting is that you follow your doctor's orders as well as see a chiropractor. Remember, because all of the tissues in your body are controlled and regulated by your nervous system, which exits through your spine, there can be no healing without your nervous system. A chiropractic adjustment can improve your nerve function.

In this light, your chiropractor has no idea what can improve after an adjustment. All he or she knows for a fact is that your body will function better after it has been adjusted. Though his or her intended result may be the removal of low-back pain through the repair of damaged, low-back muscles, you might also find that your liver begins functioning better because the same nerve that was causing you pain was also inhibiting your liver from functioning optimally. Without even realizing it, your chiropractor could make both of these problems better simply by bringing your damaged nerve back into balance. Indeed, as chiropractors, we only improve your spinal motion, which ultimately affects your nervous system. From there, your body's internal mechanisms take over and fix what they deem necessary.

Periodically I hear people boast that they have never needed a chiropractor because they have never experienced back pain. That statement tells me that the chiropractic profession has not done a good job at educating the world about its true function as a practice. Your back pain will generally go away after your spine has been adjusted, but even if you don't have pain, you still need an adjustment. We all move, and we are all under the force of gravity. And for those two reasons alone, no one is exempt from needing chiropractic care.

Lesson 4: We all need a chiropractic adjustment from time to time.

Points to Remember

1. The brain and its associated spinal cord control everything in the human body.

2. All joints are meant to move, and any lack of motion can cause joint- degenerative arthritis.

3. Chiropractic adjustments move fixated joints and improve joint motion, preventing arthritis. A properly moving joint is a happy joint.

4. Chiropractors can balance the nervous system by directly affecting the spinal cord and its nerves or by balancing the sensations being sent to the brain.

"Health is not valued till sickness comes."

Dr. Thomas Fuller

Lesson 5

Nutrition—a Jagged Little Pill?
The Truth on Vitamins

I am not the chiropractor who is constantly pushing vitamins. I first and foremost believe that your nutrition should be derived from food. Still, I have many vitamins for sale in my office. Why?

There are times when taking herbs and vitamins are absolutely necessary. I am a big believer in disease prevention, and if you have a great diet with no disease processes in your body, then you likely don't need supplementation. However, most patients who come into my office are already suffering from a disease process, and the amount of nutrients that they need to repair their bodies cannot be retrieved in enough quantity from food alone.

That being said, you need to be aware that there are a million false claims out there about the benefits of different vitamin supplements. The Internet especially has become a breeding ground for false claims in an attempt to rob you of your money. For this reason, throughout this lesson, we are going to look at the validity of some vitamins and the important role they play in keeping you healthy.

A while back, a patient of mine was tested, and his doctor determined that he had too much acid in his body. So he came to me looking for help. At the time, I had a fabulous antioxidant drink for him, but he did not want to take it because it was going to cost him $45 a month. So I gave him a recipe for an antioxidant shake that he could make at home using blended spinach as the main ingredient. After a month, he returned to me feeling better but reporting that he had spent over $150 that past month getting enough vegetables to make his shake. Needless to say, once he realized how expensive the quantity of vegetables he needed to reduce the acid in his body was going to be, he decided that he was ready to buy my antioxidant drink for $45 instead.

In addition to wanting to help my patients save money, I often suggest supplements when I encounter patients who are not able or simply refuse to eat a proper diet. Travelling salesmen and truck drivers, for instance, have little choice but to eat fast, junk food when they are on the road. On the other hand, some people just refuse to eat fruits and vegetables, even though they are not travelling. Supplementation is a must for both of these types of people.

Moreover, some sources are now reporting that the nutritional value in produce has been greatly depleted over the last 50 years due to the soil being depleted of its nutrients via fertilizers, which are used to expedite the growth and development of produce. Because of this, I have chosen to live on a farm and grow 90% of the food that I eat. I do not use pesticides or herbicides, and I grow mainly non-GMO (genetically modified organisms) seeds. My fruits and vegetables are as healthy as they can be, but even I don't get 15 servings of fruits and vegetables a day. So I take a whole-food, vegetable supplement everyday called Greens First. Days that I exercise, I take a double dose to assist my body in fighting the acid and free radicals my exercise produced, which we have talked about several times throughout this book.

As you can see, I personally live close to the earth, in that I grow a large, organic garden and eat only free-range local organic meats. I do not consume fast food on a regular basis, nor do I live off of junk food. I cook meals from scratch every day. There may be people out there who eat healthier than I do, but they are rare. My diet is about as clean as it can get, yet I still find it necessary to take vitamin supplements. The advantage for me is that because I am a healthcare provider, I know how to read through the garbage on labels and discern what truly is beneficial for my family. I have no money to waste on products that do not or cannot work.

All of that being said, there are two types of vitamin categories that I would like to talk about. The first type consists of the base vitamins that your body needs to prevent disease. I am a big proponent of preventing disease; and for that reason, I take vitamins every day, but only in forms and concentrations needed for prevention. I will tell you what I do for prevention and what I think is necessary.

I find vitamins used for the prevention of disease to be much more exciting than those used to treat a disease. For without a doubt, it is much harder to fix a problem than it is to prevent a problem. To prevent disease, I consume daily a high-quality, omega-3 oil that is extracted from fish, not from plants. I also take a vitamin D that is dissolved in oil along with a high-antioxidant, plant-based, greens supplement that has a mega dose of naturally found vitamins and minerals. Out of all of those, consuming a high antioxidant, plant-based, greens supplement is most imperative.

The second group of vitamins I want to discuss here are those vitamins that you should use for the treatment of disease. Now when it comes to this group, we have to tread lightly. No vitamin company can state or claim that one of its vitamins is a cure for a specific disease. Pharmaceutical companies spend billions of dollars doing controlled studies that allow them to state that they can actually cure a disease, but no vitamin company can afford to execute the research it would take to make such claims. For example, when I state that I will take specific vitamins to treat an infection, it is because I know through research that the vitamins I am going to take can boost my immune system. The internal workings of your body constitute the most complex and marvelous system ever created. Thus, if you can find ways to stimulate its internal power so that it can heal itself, then you can say that it really is your body that is curing the disease, not the vitamins. The vitamins will just give you the much-needed boost.

Bearing that in mind, if I have a cold, fever, sinus congestion, stomach pain, diarrhea, or just a feeling of being unwell, I will take extra vitamins in addition to those I take during my daily routine. First, I will double up on what I am already taking. On a normal day, I take three drops of vitamin D, which is 6000 units of D3. But when I don't feel well, I will take this supplement at least twice a day and maybe more. I also will take two doses of my greens supplement along with immune-boosting vitamins, such as a high-quality vitamin C or colloidal silver.

Conversations about vitamins can be very complex and often times confusing. Hence, in a quest to keep this book as simple as possible and to keep it focused on how to live longer and healthier through the prevention of disease, I will only talk about a select few vitamins and how they may assist us in our task.

If you have a specific condition such as high cholesterol, heart disease, arthritis, obesity or any other condition that vitamin supplementation can help, I suggest that you consult your vitamin specialist. This specialist could be a naturopath, a medical doctor skilled in vitamin supplementation, or any chiropractor experienced in nutrition supplementation. Don't assume that every doctor is highly skilled in the art of supplementation. This field is very complex, and heavy marketing by vitamin companies may convince doctors to sell their products even if they are not the best supplement. Such marketing might also confuse some doctors and keep them from suggesting the proper supplement, much in the same way as pharmaceutical companies have been known to influence many doctors' decisions about appropriate medication.

In addition to taking vitamins, another thing you should consider doing at least once a year is a body detoxification. I choose to perform an anti-inflammatory detox, a liver detox, and a kidney detox just after Christmas and New Year's. I do this annually because I feel that after the holidays I have abused my body by consuming too much food…especially sweets. These detox programs give my body time to catch up and start the new year feeling great.

By and large, the topic of detoxification remains greatly misunderstood—mainly because it shouldn't be called a detoxification at all. In the medical community, the term detoxification is reserved for people trying to sober up from drug abuse or for those who have sustained accidental exposure to toxic chemicals, such as mercury. The nutritional concept of detoxification is much different.

It has been discovered that certain nutrients in high concentrations can speed up the activity of specific organs or chemical reactions within organs. Detoxification of a liver, for instance, is simply giving the body excess nutrients that are known to speed up the liver, and thus increasing its ability to do its job of filtering your blood. Kidney detoxification is similar, but the nutrients you take will speed up the kidney function.

With that in mind, the detoxifications that I do yearly really just speed up my organs to flush out all of the negative substances I have ingested throughout the year, giving me a great, clean start for the next year.

So what types of nutritional supplements and detoxification products should you buy? There are many products available on the market but as I alluded to earlier not all are not created equal. I will list below the products that I personally use. However, do realize that there are other companies that make similar good quality concoctions.

```
Antioxidant Drink   ---------------Greens First
Fish Oil  (Refrigerated)-----------Metagenics EPA/DHA
Liver Cleanse   --------------------- Ultraclear PH
Anti-Inflammatory Cleanse  ----  Ultrainflam X
Kidney Cleanse    ----------------- Renagen DTX
```

Take note that these products are for prevention purposes only. When people come to my office and are experiencing a disease process, I may use any of the above products and many more. Generally people who are already sick need more help than the person who simply wants to prevent disease.

You also need to remember that I am not saying that any of these products should replace medications that you may have been taking for your condition. I do not take people off medications. That is between them and their doctor. However, it is true that any good doctor will help his or her patients remove medication from their daily routines once their symptoms and condition have improved.

Like I said earlier, food is the best form of vitamins. And with today's modern abundance of diverse foods, there should be no logical reason for you to take vitamins. However, that statement assumes that you eat the correct foods. You cannot eat prepackaged meals or snack foods and think that you are getting enough vitamins and minerals. People who refuse to eat correctly must have vitamin supplementation to compensate for the deficiencies stemming from their lacking diet.

As a logical human being, I know that there is no real reason to give any of my patients vitamin supplementation. But I cannot turn my back on the fact that many of my patients, who eat pretty good diets, still suffer undesirable symptoms, and have been greatly helped with vitamin supplementation. Likewise, I believe that I personally have one of the best diets in the world. I eat plenty of fruits, berries, vegetables, cold-water fish and local, free-range, meat products. Yet still, there have been times when I have felt fatigued around 3 or 4 p.m. The nutritional supplement Greens First cured this symptom in only a week. As long as I continue to take it, my fatigue doesn't resurface. The supplement must be supplying something that I am lacking in my diet to have such a potent physiological effect, so I take it every day and plan to continue taking it. It is a small price to pay to feel great.

When I began writing this lesson, I had no intention of listing all of the vitamin and herb products that are available on the market. There are many texts created by people more intelligent than I that can give you the specific uses for each product along with all of the pros and cons of taking those products. Truly, there are so many products on the market that it can make your head spin. To make matters worse, marketing people can do a great job at swindling uneducated patients into buying just about anything. The Better Business Bureau has a list a mile long with money-grubbing, con artists who have tried to sell snake oils by using fear tactics. Be very careful about where and from whom you buy your nutrition products. Do your own research if you question a product, and remember that the Internet is not always the best place to get your knowledge.

On occasion, I have patients come into my office with shopping bags full of vitamins that they are taking. They want my opinion on the supplements. I look at these people no differently than I look at patients who are consuming bags of prescription medications. I know that, at some point, their health has gone down the tubes and that they have been grabbing at straws to try and find help ever since. My heart goes out to these people, but I will tell you that health is rarely found at the bottom of a shopping bag full of pills. Hence, I generally tell these patients that if they want to be healthier, they need to reduce their excess vitamin intake and simply eat better.

Lesson 5: Swallowing pills won't make you healthy, even if they are vitamins.

Points to Remember

1. Better diets are preferred over taking vitamins. More vitamins are not better.

2. Supplement your food with vitamin products based on what is lacking in your diet. For example, take fish oil if you don't consume enough wild caught ocean going cold-water fish.

3. A whole-food, high antioxidant drink can be very beneficial.

4. Beware of people selling the new miracle vitamin. Research the product, and make your own decision before you waste your money.

"If a man is to live, he must be all alive, body, soul, mind, and heart."

Thomas Merton

Lesson 6

Don't Worry; Be Happy

Life is good, but life is more than your physical body. You might be as healthy as a horse, but if everything else in your life sucks, than what's the point? You must also be concerned with your mental attitude and emotional stability—not to mention all of the other facets of your life, including your spirituality, family life, social life, financial wellbeing, life's purpose and even sexual fulfillment. Of course, all of those facets are important to living well, but most exist outside the scope of this book. I do find it fitting, however, to talk about your emotional and mental wellbeing, since both of those states of being can be dramatically related to your diet.

Please remember that this book is focused on living well and living long, so before I get into how diet can affect your brain chemistry and moods, I must talk about an observation that I have made from treating thousands of patients. Every time I treat an elderly patient who is aging very slowly and has little to no elderly diseases, I make a point to talk to them so as to try and determine the secret to their success. I have heard a lot of different answers to that question. Some say, "I drink two glasses of wine every day." Others might say, "I try not to eat too much," or, "I walk every day." All of these are important things to keep in mind if you wish to age gracefully. However, more often than not, the common thread I see in these long-living patients is a specific type of mental attitude and life purpose. Let me put it this way: People who find reasons to live as well as an overall purpose for their lives are generally happier...or at least that is the way it appears to me.

Happier people also seem to have better health. I personally believe that each life must have an individualized purpose and that if a person is not expressing that purpose with their life, then life will try to take them out of existence. How many times have we seen people get sick and die after their spouses pass away or after someone retires? We were not meant to sit on the sofa and watch television all day. We must have a purpose.

People who know their purpose have a spring in their step and a smile on their face. Their mental attitude is pleasant and strong. This sets the stage for proper brain and body chemistry. A purposeful, pleasing, mental attitude backed with proper diet, exercise, water consumption, and chiropractic care will lead you to many years of happy occupancy on this earth.

Patients who constantly grumble about all of the problems in the world and always choose to be pessimistic seem to be more sick and age more rapidly than their higher-spirited peers. Are they pessimistic because they are sick, or are they sick because they are pessimistic? If I had to choose which of these situations are more plausible, I would say that they are sick because they are pessimistic. Patients who are always in a great mood rarely seem to get sick, and when they do catch a cold or have low back pain, they seem to improve more quickly than those patients who choose to be pessimistic. There is no doubt in my mind that people's mental attitudes have a great deal to do with them aging slowly and warding off sickness. That is why I have included it in this book under Lesson 6. And yes, your diet can have a dramatic influence on your moods and overall outlook on life.

Before we can get very far in this discussion, we must consider proper brain chemistry. This can be a twisted and difficult conversation; however, it is a conversation that I often have with my patients and find appropriate to elaborate upon here.

When it comes to moods, the brain generally functions with three basic chemicals: dopamine, serotonin, and oxytocin. The anatomy of the male brain is hardwired for the effects of dopamine, and when it is deprived of this chemical, men often get depressed and feel like life is not worth living. On the other hand, the female brain needs serotonin and oxytocin to be happy. Without these two neurochemicals being secreted in the female brain, happiness is nothing more than a pipe dream.

Regardless of whether you are a man or woman, if I injected you with dopamine you would feel powerful and in control. In fact, you would feel like you were the boss in the room and that everyone should listen to what you have to say. This mood is generally very pleasing to men; hence, if we reduce the levels of dopamine in men, most will feel very depressed. Women, however, are not driven by the sensation of a powerful personality. Therefore, mood disorders in women normally are not due to dopamine deficiencies.

Assuming again that you are healthy, if I injected you with serotonin and oxytocin, you would feel loved, cared for, and content. Overall, these two hormones will produce the warm, fuzzy feeling in you that makes you feel like you are supported in life and loved by everyone. The average female brain interprets these feelings as very enjoyable, leaving the woman feeling depressed if she is deprived of these two chemicals.

With this understanding of brain chemistry and how it differs between men and women, it becomes clearer as to why men and women act the ways they do. We are equal, but we are very different. Everyone wants to feel rewarded; therefore we will all do activities that give our brains positive enforcement. Men simply will do activities that stimulate the secretion of dopamine, while women will do activities that stimulate the secretions of serotonin and oxytocin.

This is a great junction to make another key point. Some men love the feelings evoked by the brain's release of serotonin and oxytocin. Likewise, many women may love the rush of dopamine. We all have different variations in our needs to feel happy, and our need for different levels of serotonin, oxytocin, and dopamine are no different. Rather, this is just one of the many ways in which you and I are unique. So when I say that a man enjoys the rush of dopamine, I am not speaking as a sexist at all; I am speaking from a place of generality. Just as some women enjoy the feeling of dominance that dopamine affords them, so some men need the comfort and contentment that is fostered by serotonin and oxytocin.

To assist you in stimulating these positive brain chemicals, there are some foods that seem to help. These foods offer the building blocks for the production of the neurochemicals dopamine and serotonin; however, you should know that your mental fixation and thoughts ultimately regulate and determine your brain's production of these neurochemicals. I will explain more about this later, but first let's take a look at the ways in which different types of food can serve as building blocks for the production of your brain's positive hormones.

The building block of dopamine is the amino acid tyrosine. If you want to help stimulate the production of dopamine, you can consume the amino acid supplement tyrosine or you can eat foods that are naturally high in tyrosine. Seeds and nuts, like almonds and pumpkin seeds, as well as fruits like blueberries, avocados, and bananas can help stimulate dopamine levels. Some research even states that high-protein foods like meat and dairy can trigger dopamine production. So if you are feeling a little blue due to a dopamine deficiency, you can help stabilize your moods by taking tyrosine supplements or eating the foods listed above.

In addition, you should take into account the fact that dopamine generally declines as you age. Therefore, it is imperative that you find ways to slow the decline in dopamine production if you wish to feel happy as you age. Eating well and not losing sight of your purpose throughout the years are two of the biggest ways that you can do this. If you choose to not be intentional about keeping your dopamine production from slowing down, depression will be sure to occur.

On the other hand, if you decide that you need to correct a deficiency in serotonin, you can either do so by taking a tryptophan or 5-HTP supplements, or you can seek to eat foods that are rich in tryptophan. Such foods include tofu, black-eyed peas, walnuts, almonds, and roasted pumpkin seeds. You can also find tryptophan in warm milk and turkey.

Completely unlike dopamine and serotonin, oxytocin is mainly secreted through the stimulation of physical touch. In other words, your brain secretes oxytocin when someone you love touches you. The same is true for your spouse if you were to rest your hand on his or her shoulder or caress his or her back. We are highly social creatures, and we crave human contact. If we get that contact, we feel loved, causing our chances of developing a mood disorder to be much less. Conversely, if we are denied touch, mental disorders can arise. So touch your loved ones the way they want to be touched.

Now let's talk about controlling your thoughts. Patients who regularly take anti-depressant medications are often told by their doctors that they have a chemical imbalance. In general, most doctors treat such imbalances through certain types of medication that can stimulate production of the deficient chemical. This may be true; however, I would argue that we have forgotten the control we have as human beings over our own brain chemistry. Let me give you an example that I sometimes give to my patients.

If I asked you to close your eyes and mentally picture being trapped, abandoned, alone, depressed, and possibly abused, your dopamine, serotonin, and oxytocin levels would plummet through the floor, and you would interpret the feelings triggered by their absence as depression or anxiety. On the other hand, if I got you to mentally picture yourself receiving a compliment from the person you love most in the world, winning the lottery, being on vacation, or sitting in the mountains by a peaceful stream, you would get a natural heavy dose of dopamine and serotonin, making you feel happy and as though your life has meaning.

What does this mean? I contend that it means you have control over your brain chemistry, and therefore, over your brain's dopamine, serotonin, and oxytocin production. After all, it was your brain that restricted and released the production of those chemicals all by itself without the use of medication when you chose to think upon different negative or positive scenarios, wasn't it? You do have control. You can change your moods without always needing medication. Now please understand that I would never belittle your struggle by stating that you never need medication, but you need to realize that becoming a slave to the chronic use of medication offers little hope to living a happy life.

Thus, learn to fixate your thoughts on positive things and less on the negative side of life. By doing so, you will be on a better path to fixing mood disorders and mental illnesses in your life. Surely at any given time both great and sad things are happening in the world around you, and for the most part, you and I have very little control over those things. This lack of control can make us feel helpless. But choosing to focus on the helpless and evil side of life will gain no one anything, aside from possible hurt. Learn to see the good in people and in life, and you will reap the benefits of feeling happier.

Likewise, it has been known for a long time that stress can kill you by weakening your immune system and leaving you susceptible to harmful infections. It can cause excessive plaque to build up in your arteries and thereby increase your chances of a heart attack. And even worse, mental stress can do these destructive things and more. But it doesn't have to be this way.

People believe that they have no choice in how they respond to stressful situations, but such a belief is not true. You are the controller of your mind, and you can control how you react to life's situations. Choose a better reaction and live healthier and longer.

Science also has proven that your emotional state can directly influence your genetic code, expressing genes based on how you feel. Hence, emotions and having a purpose in life can dramatically change your physiology and affect your sense of wellbeing. For those of you who doubt this statement, ask yourself if you have ever been scared to the point that all of the color left your face, or anxious enough that your face turned red. All of us have experienced these changes, and the accompanying feelings are due to the constriction and dilation of blood vessels in our faces. But our change in blood flow was not due to a temperature change in the room; it was provoked by our emotions. Such observations prove that your emotions can change your physiology.

So let's not kid ourselves. If our emotions can change the flow of blood to our faces, can they not also change the rate of blood flow to our livers, kidneys, spleens, or stomachs? Of course they can! We have known for decades that emotions can change the flow of blood to a person's brain and stomach in order to create a sensation of anxiety or "butterflies" in a person's stomach. But if the negative feelings we experience can rob blood flow from our organs, what will positive emotions do? Thinking positive, powerful thoughts that cultivate a sense of personal belonging can enhance the body's ability to heal itself, improve organ function, and slow aging. These are all truths that should not be taken lightly. Live happier, and you will live longer.

Case in point, the 2005 Archives of General Psychiatry conducted a controlled study on the inhibiting effects that negative thinking and emotional frustration can inflict upon the human body's ability to heal itself. To conduct the study, researchers inflicted two different groups of married couples with individual blisters.

The researchers allowed one group to heal naturally, while ordering the other group to spend their time arguing about past problems they had experienced in their relationships. At no surprise to me, the couples who argued healed 40% slower than the group who healed naturally, thus proving that bad emotions and frustration do slow down the human body's ability to heal. Like we discussed in the previous lesson, your body is constantly healing itself—and not just skin lesions or other things that your eyes can see. At any time, your body is also healing damaged tissues inside you that you cannot see. If you choose to slow down your body's healing processes by regularly dwelling on negative thoughts, you will have more chronic health problems and possibly even die early.

From a personal standpoint, I can tell you that after treating thousands of patients, I know for a fact that those who struggle with their health often have a sense of displacement with regards to their family and community. They feel like no one cares about their wellbeing, so they give up hope. And as a result, their health fades. Sadly, this is a type of mental disorder that is self-inflicted. It is easier to stay home all day and watch television than it is to go to work, school, church or your local hospital to volunteer. But while it may be easier, it is not the right way to act. Life that is lived well is a full-time job. It takes effort to eat well, exercise, go to your chiropractor and be involved in your community. But this effort is the only thing that will ensure you a great life. A passive life is not worth living. But an active life—one you intentionally and vigorously work at with all of your heart, soul, and body—is.

People who live long and healthy often state that they have a reason for being alive. These individuals are often our fellow citizens who are committed to a charity, church or some other greater humanitarian good. They feel that their life has meaning, and that feeling drives them to live a long and healthy life spent pursuing that meaning.

Do you have a passion that is worth committing to? Do you have loved ones who are special enough to you that you are willing to dedicate your time, effort and love to them? Are you a part of an organization that is engaged in activities whose legacy will live well after you are gone from this planet? Do you have a greater sense of belonging to the world or a creator?

You need to feel like you belong to a helpful, larger group—a feeling that, for the most part, has been lost in our modern-day, busy life. You must try to get the sense of community back into your life at all costs. Find people who think like you and are on a similar mission. They can be a part of a church, foundation, non-profit movement, rotary club or a well-organized profession. I personally belong to a rotary club that has a mission greater than any one individual could accomplish, and that gives me the sense that my work, money and time have an effect that will far outlive me.

I also find happiness in being a part of the struggling profession of chiropractic. This is because the constant struggle chiropractors are currently facing is forcing us to bond together to prove to the majority of the population that we have something to offer the world. The unity found in joining together with my other colleagues in a common fight for chiropractic allows me to have a deeper sense of purpose. I am a part of the solution rather than a part of the problem. What a great place to be!

All of this community and social involvement gives me purpose and joins me together with like-minded individuals. The people in my social circles are my community. They are my family and they give me the motivation to persist on. Find your passion for life, and you will have a deeper sense of life-purpose. I can promise you that you will be happier and healthier for you effort.

Indeed, we *do* need the building blocks of tryptophan and tyrosine for the production of serotonin and dopamine, respectively. But as stated earlier, having the building blocks of these neurochemicals is only half of the battle. We also must learn to focus on the good things in life, choosing to remember the good times with our spouses and not the disappointments. If our brains were focused on the positive, I am convinced that it would be very difficult for us to develop mental illnesses.

Lesson 6: Eat to stay happy.

Points to Remember

1. Eat foods high in tyrosine and tryptophan to help stimulate the neurochemicals dopamine and serotonin.

2. Focusing on negative thoughts reduces the amount of serotonin and dopamine secreted by the brain.

3. Focusing on the positive aspects of life increases the brain's secretion of dopamine and serotonin.

4. We are social creatures, and we need to be touched by people we love to help stimulate our brain's secretion of oxytocin.

"Eat healthy, sleep well, breath deeply, move harmoniously."

Jean-Pierre Barral

Lesson 7

The Final Lesson—Sleep

It was extremely difficult to determine where to put this lesson within this book. I have tried to place each lesson in order of importance from greatest to least as they relate to your quest of staying healthy and living longer, but where could I put sleep? Sleeping is a very important function for health and could just as easily have been listed as the first lesson in this book. Nevertheless, because sleeping is more passive and a simpler concept to discuss than the previous lessons, I decided to place it last. All of that being said, most health books don't even mention sleep. So why is sleep so important?

While you are sleeping, your body relaxes and rejuvenates itself. Damaged tissues such as cuts, scrapes, and bruises heal the most while you sleep. And more importantly, your body heals the tissues that you can't see while you sleep.

Everyday your body ruptures blood vessels, loses skin cells, and damages the lining of your stomach. These injuries receive the most healing from your body when you are asleep. That is why you may have noticed that healing cuts often seem better after you wake up in the morning. Conversely, individuals who do not sleep well often seem to heal slower than individuals who sleep normally.

According to the book *Growth Hormone: Reversing Human Aging Naturally*, the body secretes growth hormone while it's asleep. Growth hormone has been called the fountain of youth because higher secretions of it within the human brain can significantly lessen the effects of aging, including weight gain, muscle loss, memory loss and even skin wrinkles.

Of course, anxiety, poor eating habits, abnormal work schedules and stress can all result in decreased amounts of sleep. I am not a stranger to these stressors, but we have to see past these problems and focus on their solutions. To put it simply, you will feel healthier and think clearer if you get enough sleep.

Let me give you a few tips to help you sleep better. First, you should not eat anything three to four hours before bedtime. Digesting a heavy meal before bed will not allow your body to fully rest and may even cause indigestion.

Secondly, you should never read or watch television in bed, especially the news. Watching exciting or stressful shows or reading suspenseful novels can only hinder a calm night's sleep. The bed should be classically conditioned for sleep. If you do other activities, especially stressful activities in bed, your brain will associate the bed with everything except sleep. Once you have your brain conditioned that your bed is where you sleep, you will discover that you get sleepy the instant your head hits the pillow.

"So how much sleep is enough?" you might ask.

That is a difficult question to answer. Each person requires different amounts of sleep to function well. However, we do know for a fact that no full-grown adult needs ten hours of sleep. Nor can a full-grown adult function properly on five hours. As a general rule, adults should get between seven and eight hours of uninterrupted sleep each night. Seven to eight hours will give your body an ample amount of time to repair damaged tissues and for your brain to secrete human growth hormone.

Sleeping is a simple task, but that does not mean that it is not a vitally important one. However, if you get enough sleep along with implementing the other lessons discussed throughout this book, you most certainly will be healthier and age slower.

Lesson 7: Sleeping beauty.

Points to Remember

1. Your body heals itself the most while you sleep.

2. Your brain secretes growth hormone mainly while you sleep.

3. A higher level of growth hormone reduces the signs of aging.

4. To improve sleeping, do not eat three to four hours before bed. Also refrain from reading or watching television in bed.

"Be yourself and think for yourself; and while your conclusions may not be infallible, they will be nearer to right than the conclusions forced on you by those who have a personal interest in keeping you in ignorance."

Elbert Hubbard

Pulling It All Together

So the real question still remains: Can we prevent our families and ourselves from dying young? Do we have any hope of changing our fates? Can we alter our outcomes if we change our unhealthy ways? I believe we can.

Sickness has always been around. In the past, people were dying of strokes, heart attacks, and infectious diseases. But if you did not have these terminal conditions, the general population was healthy and well. As a doctor that deals with thousands of patients a year, I will tell you that it is getting more and more rare to see a person who is actually well. Almost everyone is dealing with some nuisance of a condition that requires medication or sheer willpower to suffer through perpetual symptoms. I know that the natural order of things is to be well, yet even patients who seem healthy at first glance are dealing with upset stomachs, depression, sleep disturbances, anxiety, skin rashes...the list goes on. We have entered into an era where it is normal to experience sickness. This phenomenon is relatively new, and I am happy to say it is avoidable.

With the exception of a few individual people, we are all born into perfect health. Therefore, it has been our lifestyles that have created our sicknesses. If we bear this in mind then, we should be able to recover our bodies by reverting back to better lifestyles. But what can we do?

This book has been written to show you that the elusive nature of wellness does not have to stay a mystery. Health can be yours as long as you do what is necessary for your body to self-regulate and heal.

The healthcare field is a trillion dollar industry in the United States of America alone. This fact makes one wonder if our society is truly seeking cures for human disease or simply teaching people to spend their money in a quest to stay alive.

The current mission of the medical field for dealing with disease is not to cure anything but to help you find a way to live with disease. When we go to the doctor, we don't get our allergies cured; we get shots and medications to help alleviate our symptoms. Likewise, people with arthritis are not getting cured, they simply are being taught to deal with the pain. We aren't finding cures for high blood pressure; we are taking pills to dilate our blood vessels and thereby reduce the pressure. But what if there really were cures for these ailments? What if all we had to do was eat better, drink better, think better and move better? Are all of the conditions that plague human society preventable? These are all great questions.

I am not naive to the fact that some diseases are genetic and that some conditions, like broken bones and head trauma, truly need medical intervention. But we have to realize that the healthcare industry has changed its focus from health care to disease care. Because of this, the majority of the population focuses their time, effort, and dollars on the management of disease rather that the cure or prevention of it—which would be true health care. Capitalism has ruined a profession that was initially altruistic in nature. Money has become the new goal of the healthcare industry, not health.

Mass media, especially the Internet, has bombarded us with so many "health drinks," "healthy snacks," and "healthy tips" that we have forgotten to think for ourselves. Scientists have tried to break down food into vitamins, minerals, and nutrients rather than teach people how to eat real food. By and large, we have become so dependent on scientific information that we believe a protein bar is healthier than an egg, or that milk formula is better than mother's milk.

But don't fret! There is a wave of people starting to fight back, and their fight is creating a ripple in the economics of healthcare. Ultimately, the just will win. There will eventually be some sanity placed back in healthcare because this small-yet-powerful, underground movement is growing and becoming more vocal. It is a strong mixture of scientists, chiropractors, naturopathic doctors, medical doctors and highly-vocal citizens. Slowly, by teaching our kids to drink water instead of sodas and to eat local, natural, and pesticide-free food, we are returning to sanity. Finally exercise is becoming more popular, and we are realizing that stress not only kills the mind, but also the body. We will win because we are on the right side.

There are nearly seven billion people on this planet, and every one of them has cells that are mutating into cancer. Yet their bodies are isolating those cells and destroying them. By killing those cancer cells, they are inhibiting them from growing into tumors and spreading throughout their bodies. A disease-care model doesn't care about the destruction of early cancer cells. It only seeks to shrink and remove them once they have become a threat to a person's life. A true healthcare system would be more concerned with keeping the body's natural mechanisms that detect and destroy early cancer cells working at their optimum. Your body truly does have the ability to heal itself, but it needs your help. Proper diet, exercise, water consumption, and lifestyle can keep it operating efficiently. To be sure, preventing diseases, especially cancer, is a much nicer and more humane method of dealing with diseases than undergoing their treatments.

Whenever I ask my patients which is healthier—butternut squash or pizza pockets— they always get the answer correct. We are innately smart, but we do stupid things in our quest for convenience, despite the fact that our convenient lives are killing us even while we are still young.

Staying healthy is neither elusive nor difficult. We do not need experts to tell us what is healthy and what is not. All we have to do is use our brains and show a little commitment.

There are only a few things that we must do to stay well and prevent the majority of diseases, but still we act as if it is difficult. The majority of things listed throughout this book are simple procedures, such as installing water filters on your showerhead and kitchen sink. Once you install the systems, you need not think about them again for a year. How simple is that?

I have never been a radical person, but because I am so healthy, my patients believe that I must be some kind of health nut. I must admit that I am far from it. I do not perform extreme exercises and I occasionally even partake of fast food. But as you hopefully have seen throughout this book, life does not have to be extreme in order to live well. If you eat fast food once or twice a month, it will not shorten your life. On the flip side, if you eat fast food several times a week, you are heading down the path of destruction and disease. I do not teach a life of denial because it is not necessary to eliminate all of your favorite foods or to become an exercise freak. A life of common sense and moderation is all that is needed to live well.

Now, just in case you haven't already noticed, nowhere in this book have I mentioned the use of tobacco. I didn't find that topic necessary because I can't think of a person in his or her right mind who would suggest that smoking is okay. Even still, when I go on vacation to the Caribbean, I thoroughly enjoy smoking a nice cigar. It's fine! One cigar once a year will never kill you; just like one soda a month will not shorten your life. It is smoking or drinking sodas daily that will cause you to die prematurely.

Living well and living healthy is not complicated and we need not make it more complicated than necessary. We are the only animals on this planet who strive to make our lives more difficult than they need to be. Moderate exercises, increased water consumption, limited junk food, and a positive, mental attitude are all that is needed for a healthy lifestyle. Stop looking for quick weight-loss pills and diets. You don't need meal replacements. You need healthy meals.

Throughout this book, we have seen that many conditions we expect in life prove to actually be preventable. If you choose to follow the simple lessons laid out in this book, you will experience a healthier and happier life. I would love to see every person get back to living well instead of fighting through life, chasing one symptom after another. I especially want this for today's children.

Children do not have fully-formed minds, nervous systems, and bodies. Their genetics are not even as fully cemented as a full-grown adult's. If we were to get our children to live healthier lifestyles, we could have a dramatic impact on their futures and the future of the world.

Even so, I often hear parents complain, "But my child won't eat fruits and vegetables."

Step up, and be a parent, not their friend. Children will eat what they are told to eat if you start them at a young age. Children will also eat what they see their parents eating. Besides that, no person will choose to starve when there is food in front of them. Sure, if you give your kids an option to eat real food or pizza pockets, they might choose the pizza pocket. So don't give them the option. Take control of their health. Be your children's parent. Be their leader.

In my quest to get people to eat better, I often hear, "But Dr. Short, healthy food is too expensive. I can't afford salmon and organic vegetables." This is when I know I will have my work cut out for me.

According to the U.S government's economics in 1900, the average American household spent 40% of their income on food. Today, that average is between 6% and 8%. We are a culture that would rather buy cheap, unhealthy food so that we can save money for a new cell phone. Is a bigger house more important than being healthy? Do we really need that extra car more than we need better food? We have lost our way. We have distorted our priorities. We need to spend our money on our health and on the health of our children.

The long and short of it is this: You create your health. Likewise, you create your sicknesses. There are only a few exceptions to this statement, like people born with genetic conditions and unusual, genetic predispositions (like genetic-style cancer). But these situations are relatively rare. For the most part, you earn your life—be it health or sickness. It is the collection of all of the things that you have done that have led you to where you are. Before you can truly begin the process of healing yourself, you first must take ownership of the conditions you have created.

The body has an amazing power to heal and regenerate. Start now, and you can live a long, healthy life. I want to be a part of the new health revolution. I want to help. Let's band together and live out the principles taught in this book. Then we will not die young.

Appendix A

Foods to Eat

Fruits and Vegetables

-Green, leafy vegetables (chard, turnip greens, beet greens, and kale)
-Asparagus
-Tomatoes in as many different colors as possible
-Squash from a variety of different colors (zucchini, yellow crook neck, etc.)
-Winter squash (butternut, spaghetti, acorn)
-Peppers in as many different varieties and colors as you can find
-Okra
-Beets in a variety of different colors
-Carrots
-Eggplant
-Onions and garlic
-Fresh herbs
-Berries of all varieties (not canned whenever possible; frozen is okay)
-All fruit with a variety of colors (not canned whenever possible)

Meats

-Chicken, turkey, duck (organically and/or locally grown whenever possible)
-Beef (organically and/or locally grown whenever possible)
-Pork (organically and/or locally grown whenever possible)
-Fish and shellfish (saltwater fish is better than freshwater fish, and wild-caught is preferred over farm-raised)

-Eggs (organically and/or locally grown whenever possible)

-Processed meat (bologna, salami, pepperoni, etc. should be consumed in small amounts and less often than whole meats).

Note: Please read the ingredients listed on the back label of processed meats since some contain a lot of preservatives and additives while others may only contain whole ingredients. The ingredients could vary greatly one brand from the next.

Foods to Avoid or Consume Sparingly

-Soda
-Store-bought cookies
-Candy
-Potato or corn chips
-Canned food
-Frozen dinners
-Premade pizza or pizza pockets
-Pop tarts
-Cereals, especially those marketed to children
-Cereal bars
-Boxed macaroni and cheese
-Foods with added dyes, preservatives, and chemicals

Appendix B

Health Questionnaire

Please answer the following questions before you start an elimination diet and then again after you have been on the elimination diet for three to four weeks. You must rate your answers on a scale from 1-10. If the question describes how you feel and your symptoms are severe, rate yourself as a 10. If the question does not apply to you, circle 0.

1. I often feel disproportionately bloated after a meal, even when I did not eat enough of the meal to feel bloated.

0   1   2   3   4   5   6   7   8   9   10

2. I often notice that I am irritable after I eat certain foods.

0   1   2   3   4   5   6   7   8   9   10

3. I get headaches often.

0   1   2   3   4   5   6   7   8   9   10

4. I constantly have either constipation or diarrhea.

0   1   2   3   4   5   6   7   8   9   10

5. My skin feels older, thinner, or too wrinkled for my age.

0   1   2   3   4   5   6   7   8   9   10

6. I have a lot of joint pain.

0   1   2   3   4   5   6   7   8   9   10

7. My energy is very low, and I feel tired all of the time.

0 1 2 3 4 5 6 7 8 9 10

8. I have trouble concentrating.

0 1 2 3 4 5 6 7 8 9 10

9. My bowel movements or urine smell excessively strong.

0 1 2 3 4 5 6 7 8 9 10

10. I am constantly belching or have excessive bowel gas.

0 1 2 3 4 5 6 7 8 9 10

Total score: _____

The maximum score is 100, and the minimum is 0. If you see your score reduce dramatically after doing an elimination diet, it is very possible that you have food intolerances.

Appendix C

Things to Avoid during an Elimination Diet

Dairy products: Milk, heavy cream, half-and-half, coffee whitener (creamer), whipping cream, butter, cream cheese, yogurt, sour cream, butter milk, cottage cheese, all types of cheese, ice cream, frozen yogurt, and any cream-based salad dressings.

Milk products are hidden in many types of food, so you must read ingredient labels. There may be names that can be used to hide the fact that dairy exists in a product. These names include milk solids, processed cheese, whey or whey protein, and casein. To be on a strict elimination diet, you must remove these products.

Wheat products: Bread, cereals, cream of wheat, pancakes, waffles, crackers, pasta, bread crumbs, cakes, cookies, corn bread, pies, pizza, oats, oatmeal, honey buns, batter-fried foods, and thickened sauces such as gravy, soy sauce, and most barbeque sauces.

Reading labels will also reveal the presence of wheat in different food products with terms like enriched flour, bleached flour, wheat flour, white flour, spelt flour, durum wheat, semolina flour, gluten, or wheat protein.

Corn products: Corn, cream corn, tortillas, nachos, corn chips, Doritos, corn bread, corn meal, corn flakes, corn starch, corn syrup, sodas, as well as gravy and sauces thickened with corn starch.

Corn is one of those things that is easy to stay away from until you discover that corn byproducts are in just about everything. The ingredient names to watch out for are cornstarch, corn meal, maize, corn syrup, and high fructose corn syrup.

Eggs: Eggs, omelets, cakes, cookies, breads, French toast, pancakes, waffles, mayonnaise, and salad dressings.

By eliminating most foods containing wheat, dairy, and corn you will automatically eliminate most of your exposure to eggs. Nevertheless, if they are present in a food product, they may be listed as eggs, egg solids, egg whites, egg yolks, or egg protein.

Soy: Soy sauce, edamame (soy beans), tofu, soymilk, vegetarian meat substitutes (veggie burgers and hot dogs), and most oriental foods.

Soy by itself is easy to remove from your diet until you realize that it is used as filler in many foods. It is found in foods under the hidden names of soy protein and soy lecithin.

Appendix D

Commitment to Health

I _____ (print name) am committed to health. I know that the power to be healthy exists inside my body and that it can only be manifested by my actions. Good foods, good water, proper exercise, chiropractic treatments, and other actions mentioned in this book can dramatically improve my health. Abusing my body with poor diet, dehydration, and lack of movement will only manifest sickness. I am in control, and only I can heal my body through my actions.

I sign this document to show my commitment to being healthier and happier. I do not take this commitment lightly, and by my signature below, I dedicate my full attention to unleashing the power within my body to living happier, healthier, and with passion. I promise to spread these principles to all of mankind in a joint effort to change the world for the better. If I don't do it, who will?

_____ (Signature)

_____ (Date)

Quoted and Suggested Readings

Batmanghelidj, F. *Your Body's Many Cries for Water*. 3rd ed. Brisbane, Queensland: Global Health Solutions, Inc., 2008.

Bowden, Jonny, and Stephen Sinatra. *The Great Cholesterol Myth: Why Lowering Your Cholesterol Won't Prevent Heart Disease— and the Statin-Free Plan that Will*. Beverly, MA: Fair Winds Press, 2012.

Bowthorpe, Janie A. *Stop the Thyroid Madness: A Patient Revolution Against Decades of Inferior Thyroid Treatment*. Rev. ed. Fredericksburg, TX: Laughing Grape Publishing, LLC, 2012.

Brostoff, Jonathan, and Linda Gamlin. *Food Allergies and Food Intolerance: The Complete Guide to Their Identification and Treatment*. 3rd ed. Rochester, VT: Healing Arts Press, 2000.

Jamieson, James, L. E. Dorman, and Valerie Marriott. *Growth Hormone: Reversing Human Aging Naturally*. 5th ed. St. Louis, MO: J. Jamieson, 1997.

Kingsolver, Barbara, Steven L. Hopp, and Camille Kingsolver. *Animal, Vegetable, Miracle: A Year of Food Life*. New York: Harper Perennial, 2007.

Lipton, Bruce H. *The Biology of Belief: Unleashing the Power of Consciousness, Matter & Miracles*. New York: Hay House, Inc., 2008.

Mancini, Fabrizio. *The Power of Self-Healing*. New York: Hay House, Inc., 2012.

Pollan, Michael. *In Defense of Food: An Eater's Manifesto*. New York: Penguin Books, 2008.

Simpson, Kathryn R. *Overcoming Adrenal Fatigue: How to Restore Hormonal Balance and Feel Renewed, Energized, and Stress Free*. Oakland, CA: New Harbinger Publications, Inc., 2011.

Talbott, Shawn. *The Cortisol Connection: Why Stress Makes You Fat and Ruins Your Health—And What You Can Do about It*. 2nd ed. Ann Arbor, MI: Sheridan Books, 2007.

www.ingramcontent.com/pod-product-compliance
Lightning Source LLC
Chambersburg PA
CBHW060419290526
45791CB00002B/825